Essential Psychology for Nurses and Other Health Professionals

Understanding how individuals function psychologically in health and illness is vital to providing appropriate care for all patients and clients. With this in mind, **Graham Russell** has written a text for students in nursing and other health professions which examines key psychological concepts and shows clearly how they apply in everyday practice.

Part one explains the basis of individual psychology and how 'life events' impact on how we perceive ourselves and others too. Part two focuses on reactions to change, challenging events and loss, with particular emphasis on the nature and causes of emotional states such as anxiety, depression, anger and grief. Part three looks at key issues for health promotion, including why patients seek (or fail to seek) help and what influences compliance and non-compliance with advice from health professionals. Part four examines the links between psychological factors and physical well-being, with particular reference to stress, the cardiovascular and immune systems, and pain.

The book is also designed to develop the reader's self-awareness both in general terms and in the context of being a health care professional. The concluding chapter takes a unique look at how clinical judgements and decisions are made by generating and testing hypotheses.

Clinical scenarios and examples are used throughout to demonstrate how psychology may be applied to practice across a wide range of situations, in both hospital and community settings. Learning outcomes and self-test questions have also been included to help readers check their understanding at each stage. *Essential Psychology for Nurses and Other Health Professionals* is therefore an ideal introduction to psychological concepts for all those studying the subject for the first time.

Graham Russell is a Senior Lecturer in Health Psychology at Plymouth University and a qualified nurse.

Essential Psychology for Nurses and Other Health Professionals

Graham Russell

ROUTLEDGE

LONDON AND NEW YORK

First published 1999
by Routledge
11 New Fetter Lane, London EC4P 4EE

Simultaneously published in the USA and
Canada
by Routledge
29 West 35th Street, New York,
NY 10001

© 1999 Graham Russell

Typeset in Janson and Futura by
Keystroke, Jacaranda Lodge,
Wolverhampton

Printed and bound in Great Britain by
Creative Print & Design (Wales), Ebbw
Vale

*British Library Cataloguing in Publication
Data*
A catalogue record for this book is
available from the British Library

*Library of Congress Cataloging in
Publication Data*
Russell, Graham,
    Essential Psychology for Nurses and
Other Health Professionals / Graham
Russell.
    p.   cm.
    Includes bibliographical references and
index.
    1. Clinical health psychology.
2. Patients–Psychology.
3. Nursing–Psychological aspects.
4. Psychology. 5. Nurses. I. Title.
[DNLM: 1. Psychology nurses'
instruction. 2. Patient Care–psychology
nurses' instruction. 3. Health
Promotion. 4. Patient Compliance–
psychology. 5. Allied Health Personnel.
WY 87R963e 1999]
R726.7.R87 1999
616.89—dc21
DNLM/DLC
for Library of Congress   98–36107
CIP

ISBN 0-415-18888-1 (hbk)
ISBN 0-415-18889-X (pbk)

Contents

Part four

Part five

List of illustrations

Figures

Tables

Preface

It is the possession and application of knowledge that typically differentiates the approach of the trained and untrained nurse. It is not the ability to be practical, humane or compassionate, though even the best of intentions can be misplaced when inadequately supported by understanding.

Acknowledgements

I would like to offer warm thanks to my colleagues for their help and advice and, in particular, to Nadine Pearce, Gill McEwing and Carol Coleman. Most of all, however, I owe a special debt of gratitude to my family for their tolerance and understanding and to my wife, Ea, for her support, comments and reflections on a range of common-sense and clinical issues contained in this text.

How to use this book

In constructing this book, I have not assumed any prior knowledge of psychology or research methods, and everything covered in the text should be well within your grasp. The text is split into four main sections that are organised around the following conceptually coherent themes: Understanding ourselves and others, Reactions to change, challenging events and loss, Promoting and maintaining health, and Psycho-physiology: The relationship between mind and body. These themes are designed to offer you a broad knowledge base that embraces issues in primary, secondary and tertiary levels of care in both community and hospital based settings. To retain consistency, each chapter opens with a set of stated learning outcomes and each part concludes with a set of mini self-test questions, which you can use to test your understanding of the contents and issues.

Efforts have been made to show how psychology may be related to each of the four main branches of nursing (adult, child, mental health and learning disabilities) through the choice of material and the use of examples. At the end of each part you will find a suite of reflective scenarios, which have been constructed to afford you the opportunity to apply theory to clinical practice.

In making judgements about what to include and omit, I have drawn on my personal experience as a nurse and psychologist and consulted with colleagues to check the relevance and accuracy of the material and examples used. However, you should be aware that this text does not purport to cover all aspects of psychology, and the contents reflect my personal preferences and biases in selecting what I perceive as essential psychology for pre-registration nurses. To take a specific example, I have placed more emphasis on skills of enquiry based upon reflection and self-awareness than I have on skills of enquiry based on critical appraisal of research methodology, or on highlighting the different philosophies and approaches that guide the development and application of knowledge within the various sub-disciplines of psychology. Each approach has its merits and drawbacks, so I strongly encourage you to read widely to gain alternative insights into the issues that bind psychology and nursing together.

You will find that certain terms or words in this text are highlighted by the use of italics. This has been done to help you identify key concepts, ideas and issues. Many of these are explained in the text, but those that are not are included in the glossary of psychological and medical terms on pp. 195–208.

There are two sources of reference for the articles, journals and books cited in this text. The first is the main reference list included on pp. 209–224 and the second is the suggested reading lists that follow each of the first four sections. These may be used to supplement your knowledge base and may be helpful when you are carrying out project work or case studies.

Finally, each section contains a highlighted feature that focuses on clinical practice issues. These have been used to explore psychological issues relevant to nursing practice that might otherwise have fallen outside the scope of this text.

Part one

Understanding ourselves and others

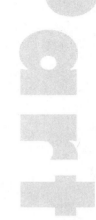

Chapter 1

Self-awareness and reflective practice

Learning outcomes

By the end of this chapter you should be able to:

- Explain why people sometimes feel uncomfortable dealing with other people's emotions.
- Describe how knowledge leads to understanding.
- Outline why reflective practice is important in the context of nursing.

Dealing with other people's emotions

Some years ago, a close friend was killed in a car crash. I was in my early twenties and was very shaken and upset by the event. Two or three days after his death, his mother contacted me and asked if I would accompany his fiancée to a bar in Oxford that he and I had regularly frequented. I agreed to do this, but felt uneasy. I hardly knew her and was unsure why she wanted to go or what she expected of me.

In the event, we sat in the bar for what seemed like a very long time and both said very little. She was clearly very upset and appeared to be in a dazed state, whilst I felt pretty useless and uncomfortable and unable to offer her much in the way of empathy or tangible support. Worse still, I remember being so focused on my own feelings of unease that I had a strong urge to escape from the situation.

Feeling uncomfortable and out of sorts when faced with serious and relatively infrequent events, such as life-threatening illness, acute mental health problems and death, is not uncommon. Parkes (1972), for example, found that recently bereaved widows frequently complained that others avoided them and were noticeably uncomfortable when talking about the deceased. Nor are nurses and other health professionals immune from such feelings. Nichols (1985), for instance, found that nurses working in a renal unit felt ill at ease and distanced themselves from patients and partners expressing negative emotions. Similarly, the Royal College of Physicians and Psychiatrists (1995) recently published a report that suggested that a lack of confidence and unease in dealing with strong emotions might be partly responsible for the many cases of moderate to severe anxiety and depression that go undiagnosed and untreated by doctors and nurses in medical settings.

In fact, there are many reasons why individuals might feel uncomfortable dealing with other people's emotions. Research by investigators such as Fenigstein et al. (1975) and Farber (1989), for example, has shown that some people have a limited awareness of their own emotional states and this may well motivate them to avoid situations that involve strong emotional responses. Similarly, Skynner and Cleese (1983) argue that children who grow up in social environments that discourage emotional expression, eventually learn to inhibit or shut off their emotions, because they feel ill at ease with them. Given this, it is not difficult to imagine that individuals socialised in this way might also seek to avoid situations that involve powerful emotions. Such explanations, however, probably explain *individual differences* in behaviour in only a small number of people, as we may assume that the majority of us mature in families that do not generally discourage the expression of emotion. So perhaps we need to look at the nature of the emotions involved and the types of event that are associated with them.

Clearly, we are not uncomfortable with powerful emotions *per se*. After all, many of us happily fall madly in love or willingly subject ourselves to high levels of fear on the latest theme park ride or gladly pay money to watch a 'weepy movie', knowing that we are going to feel sad and upset. Yet, to a large extent we have a degree of *control* over these emotions in that we can choose to avoid the theme park or terminate a relationship if our feelings start to threaten us, or walk out of the cinema if it gets too much. However, when emotions such as anger, sadness and grief are expressed by others in real, interpersonal situations, we sometimes perceive that we have little direct control over their expression or their effects on us. In addition, there are other tangible reasons why we might avoid certain types of emotion. Anger, for example, is generally regarded as socially unacceptable (particularly in women) and it often signifies the threat of physical or psychological harm that is to be avoided where possible (Berkowitz 1993). Furthermore, the powerful expression of grief and sadness may combine uneasily with the causal event to remind us of our own personal vulnerability and mortality (Bowlby 1980). In short, we are most likely to feel uncomfortable with emotion when it is negative in valence and potentially uncontrollable.

A final clue to the cause of our discomfort has already been alluded to in the previously cited report by the Royal College of Physicians and Psychiatrists. It suggests that clinical staff are reluctant to deal with emotional states such as anxiety and depression, because they feel they lack the necessary understanding and skills to deal with them competently (notably, anger often accompanies anxiety, depression and grief [Marks 1997]). Indeed, this perspective is echoed by Mead *et al.* (1997), who point out that nurses need to perceive that they are adequately trained and supported if they are to feel at ease in taking on potentially difficult interpersonal roles.

Knowledge, understanding and perception

To understand ourselves and others, we need a knowledge base that is organised in such a way that it allows us to make sense of the things that we experience. When our knowledge base is inadequate, we have difficulty understanding or perceiving what is happening and we feel uneasy. This is probably what occurred when I accompanied my friend's fiancée to the pub that night. I found her actions difficult to understand because I knew little about the processes that characterise bereavement, and I felt inadequate because I lacked the skills to handle the situation competently.

In general terms, psychologists equate understanding with perception, which is a concept that may be loosely defined as the organisation and interpretation of knowledge. Bilton *et al.* (1987) state that much of what we know, and the perceptions that flow from it, is determined by *culture*, which has been described as the DNA of society. Culture is a major determinant of how we are educated and socialised and it influences the beliefs that are filtered through society to the level of the individual (for instance, 200 years ago, you and I might well have perceived slavery as part of the natural order of things). Despite the influence of culture, however, each individual retains a unique perception or understanding of the world, and the events that occur within it, that is a function of our particular experiences relating to education, parenting, gender, class and genetic make-up (Atkinson *et al.* 1993).

Perception is an important concept in the context of clinical practice too, because, as Kagan (1987) suggests, *our personal perceptions define both the problem and our solution to it*. To put this in perspective, imagine for a moment that you live in an isolated tribal society and awake one morning to find your brother paralysed. Your definition of the problem is shaped by your belief in the power of evil spirits to invade and enslave the body, and as you have no knowledge of medical concepts such as microbes or intra-cranial bleeding, your solution to the problem is to fetch the local witch-doctor to banish the evil spirits and restore his health.

Sometimes individual differences in perception can also lead to conflict and confusion about the causes and consequences of illness, especially when the clinician and the patient or client differ in their understanding of the condition, its prevention and treatment (Steptoe and Mathews 1984). A family doctor, for example, may try hard to persuade an under-age teenager to adopt safe sex procedures, because recent experience dealing with an HIV positive patient has reinforced her perception of risk. However, the teenager may choose to disregard the advice, because she perceives her chances of contracting the disease as remote. Similarly, conflict can arise when the nurse's perception of what is best for the patient differs from that of the physician (Benner *et al.* 1996).

Reflective practice and interpersonal skills

Knowledge only leads to understanding when we consciously reflect on how our thoughts and feelings relate to the things that we observe in others or experience ourselves. In the context of nursing, this is known as *reflective practice*, and it involves asking questions, such as, 'what am I doing and thinking, why and with what effect?' (Kagan 1987, p. 33). You may find on reflection, for example, that you are irritated by an anxious patient, because you believe she is placing excessive demands on your time, or you may find that you have been avoiding a depressed patient, because he makes you feel powerless and impotent as a nurse. This form of *self-awareness* underpins a range of *interpersonal skills* that support effective nursing practice; these include communication and listening, observation of verbal and non-verbal behaviour and planning and problem-solving. Importantly, each and every one of these skills is dependent upon reflection and understanding for their effective execution, and, by the reverse order, nursing care is impoverished when understanding is constrained by overly prescriptive rules and procedures that lead to the automatic performance of tasks.

In short, reflection leads to understanding, and the more we understand about human emotion and behaviour, the more accurate are our formulations of problems and identification of needs and the more appropriate the resulting implementation of care.

Using psychological knowledge as a skill

In reading this text, you will be building upon your existing knowledge, experiences and understanding of human emotion and behaviour. In fact, students often comment that they are surprised just how much they intuitively know when they come to study psychology formally. Unfortunately, however, the feelings and perceptions that flow from 'intuition', or partially digested knowledge, are sometimes difficult to put into words and can often be expressed only by relating them to particular circumstances or episodes (Conway *et al*. 1998). In the context of nursing practice, it is obviously desirable to communicate knowledge quickly and effectively. Studying psychology can facilitate this, by providing you with a common language with which to express ideas, and by introducing you to theories, concepts and models that help you to sift and organise information in way that is conceptually coherent. This is an essential tool in the context of clinical practice. When a group of nurses collectively *know* about concepts such as stress, learned helplessness and depression, they are readily able to communicate their thoughts and ideas and apply them to the problem in hand.

Summary

Powerful emotions, such as anger, sadness and grief, can lead to feelings of unease, when we perceive that we lack control over their expression and effects, that they pose a potential threat to us or that we lack the understanding and skills to deal with them appropriately. One of the primary skills involved in understanding emotion and behaviour is termed reflective practice, which is based on self-awareness of the links between what we know, think and feel and what we observe in others or experience ourselves.

Psychologists often refer to understanding as perception or the organisation and interpretation of knowledge, which leads to a particular way of viewing the world. We share much of our perceptions with others, but each individual retains a unique understanding of the world based on his or her particular experiences. Such individual differences in perception can lead to conflict between health professionals, patients and clients, and it is important to reflect on how our thoughts and feelings influence the actions we take.

The formal study of psychology builds on the knowledge we already possess and gives us a common language with which to communicate ideas, theories and concepts. In fact, what you will learn in the following chapters is intended to build on what you know and to encourage reflective practice through self-awareness and an enhanced knowledge of others' emotions and behaviours. In the next chapter we will set the first building block in place by exploring how a knowledge of the self-system can be applied in clinical practice.

Chapter 2

The self-system

Learning outcomes

By the end of this chapter you should be able to:

- Name the basic components that comprise the self-system.
- Outline the role that beliefs play in determining behaviour.
- Describe the role of temperaments, traits and self-schemas in individual behaviour.
- Outline the basic components of self-esteem.
- Understand the relationship between life events and changes in self-esteem.

Who and what we are

We are not born with a fully developed sense of who and what we are. Our self-perceptions are based upon a sophisticated knowledge of self that is derived from a cumulative position about our past successes and failures and a knowledge of how others generally interact with us. This body of knowledge appears to evolve sometime during the second year of life and, once developed, results in stable self-perceptions during adulthood that are altered only gradually by developmental events, such as the transition from first-year student nurse to a qualified practitioner, or sometimes more radically, by major life events, such as childbirth, unemployment, bereavement, surgery and clinical depression.

In the following section we will explore the processes that underpin the development of the self and examine how individuals may respond to events that threaten their self-concept. This will provide you with a perspective that emphasises the importance of positive feedback and nurturance during childhood and an understanding of how and why individuals react to major, negative life events with a range of reactions that span extreme anxiety to outright denial.

The term *self-system* is used to describe a complex psychological phenomenon that embraces what is more commonly referred to as the individual's self-identity or self-concept. It is a system made up of four basic components (see Figure 2.1) that play a pivotal role in how we feel about ourselves and others.

The first component, *body image*, comprises a sensory awareness of the body's boundaries and an internal 'model' of our body size and shape (Fisher 1973). This model gives us a sense of unity and physical separateness from our environment and it provides us with a fairly accurate picture of how we appear to others. However, the model is perceptual, rather than factual, and is influenced by our mood states. For example, you probably have days when you feel good about yourself and confident about the way you look, and no doubt you have days when you are dissatisfied with your body shape, weight, hair, etc. Furthermore, research shows that the model we hold of ourselves does not always match reality. For example, Fallon (1990) found that women of average weight typically overestimate their body size and shape, a misperception that is expressed in an extreme form in people suffering from anorexia nervosa (Garfinkel and Garner 1982).

The second component comprises *personality traits*, which are regarded as stable and enduring characteristics of the individual. These traits are viewed as important by psychologists, because they are assumed to provide a measure of consistency that allows us to predict individual behaviour across a wide range of situations (Atkinson *et al.* 1993). For example, we would expect someone who possesses the trait of conscientiousness to be reliable and trustworthy in most, if not all, situations.

The third component of the self-system comprises the *personal belief systems* that evolve differentially in each of us as a function of our unique personal backgrounds and experiences (Sulls and Mullen 1982). These belief systems are viewed as important, because they influence our perception of ourselves and others and the world in general. For example, individuals who believe they are capable of achieving the things they aspire to, generally do better than those who have negative self-beliefs.

The fourth component, *self-esteem*, is often referred to as the evaluative aspect of self, because self-esteem is a reflection of how we feel about ourselves. It is also treated as an affective state, because self-esteem plays a key role in determining our overall mood. This mood state remains relatively stable across situations and time, though it does fluctuate in response to transient events that lift or depress us (Harter 1985).

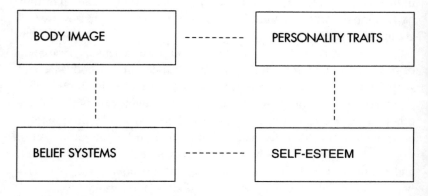

FIGURE 2.1 The four components of the self-system

The self-system and clinical practice

The self is said to be a dynamic system, because a change in a single component may have a knock-on effect on other parts of the system, which can result in major changes in the way the individual perceives his or her self. For example, surgical removal of the testes may lead to an alteration in physical body image, a self-reappraisal of sexual identity and a temporary (or perhaps enduring) loss of self-confidence and self-esteem. Similarly, an individual who suffers disfigurement, caused by serious burns to the head, face and neck, is highly likely to experience a personal crisis, if he or she is heavily reliant on appearance for self-esteem and believes that people tend to be judged by their appearance alone. In short, personal characteristics or traits, body image, personal beliefs and self-esteem are all inter-related and affect mood and behaviour.

Personal beliefs, perceptions and behaviour

The latter example illustrates how our personal beliefs may exert an influence on the way we feel about ourselves and an influence on how we may react to adverse events. However, personal beliefs also play a significant role in determining what we attend to in our environment and how we interpret the information that is gathered (Markus and Nurius 1986). For instance, it has been suggested that people prone to recurrent depression often have a negative belief system, or 'depressive set', which adversely colours their self-perceptions (Beck 1976). Take, for example, a woman passed in the street without acknowledgement by an acquaintance. If she is non-depressed, she is likely to attribute the event to her acquaintance's absent-mindedness or preoccupation rather than to some personal inadequacy. However, if she is depressed, she is more likely to reach the conclusion that she has been ignored because she is generally disliked or unworthy of others' attentions. This tendency to blame the self for failures and untoward events is an important feature of depression, and, in the latter instance, the woman's conclusion would serve only to reinforce further her already negative self-beliefs.

Whilst the latter example demonstrates the way in which personal beliefs may influence *how* we interpret information available to us, our beliefs can also exert an influence on *what* we attend to and what we ignore. Janis and Mann (1979), for example, have shown that we tend to select-out information that is at odds with our beliefs and select-in information that has the effect of confirming or bolstering them. In some instances, this may result in an unconscious distortion and oversimplification of issues and risks. Indeed, there are documented examples of this type of *cognitive bias* occurring in clinical settings. For example, kidney-donor patients provided with careful information about potential risk factors were found to make a rapid decision to donate without cautiously weighing up the relevant pros and cons. Subsequent questioning of the donors revealed that they felt morally bound to donate a kidney to a relative and, as a consequence, information about possible risks was simply ignored (Fellner and Marshall 1970; Simmons *et al.* 1973).

Such cases serve to illustrate that the patient's and health professional's beliefs can sometimes be radically different, and the nurse should not assume that the patient's perception of events will always be the same as his or her own.

Personality traits and behaviour

Traits are an important part of the individual's self-concept and may be loosely defined as a tendency to behave in a characteristic way across a broad range of situations.

Many psychologists hold the view that personality traits are laid down in childhood, as a consequence of ongoing interactions between inherited dispositions and environmental factors. Buss and Plomin (1984), for example, have shown that reliable individual differences in basic dispositions, such as concentration span, general mood, activity levels and response to environmental change, are detectable in infants as young as three months of age.

These basic dispositions, or temperaments, may be viewed as crude building blocks that interact with environmental factors to shape the individual's personality. For example, a highly active child with a poor concentration span might conceivably develop an aggressive disposition if he is situated in an environment where great emphasis is placed upon patience and academic achievement. Over a period of time, his inability to meet others' expectations might lead to repeated frustration that could eventually result in anger and aggression as a habitual response to difficult situations. Similarly, a three-month-old child who shows evidence of being uncomfortable in new environments, might conceivably develop an anxious or neurotic disposition if she is frequently moved from one child minder to another during the first year of life. In short, the traits that result from the interaction of these crude temperaments with environmental factors are formed early in life and become habitual responses to a range of situations.

Whilst psychologists cannot agree on exactly how many types of personality trait exist, recent research has indicated that five core traits underpin individual differences in personality. The 'big five', as they are sometimes referred to, comprise:

- *Neuroticism*, or the extent to which the individual worries about events and is insecure.
- *Extroversion*, or the extent to which the individual is outgoing, spontaneous and sociable.
- *Openness*, or the extent to which the individual is adventurous and liberal in his or her attitudes.
- *Agreeableness*, or the extent to which the individual is good-natured and selfless.
- *Conscientiousness*, or the extent to which the individual is reliable and trustworthy.

(McCrae and Costa 1987)

As we will see later in this text, the assumption that personality traits are relatively stable across situations has led researchers to investigate whether certain types of traits might afford individuals protection from ill-health or render them more susceptible to physical and psychological illnesses.

Personality traits are closely related to the individual's personal belief systems. For example, we might argue that the individual portrayed earlier in Beck's scenario has a depressive trait that is inextricably tied to her negative self-beliefs. Similarly, a man scoring high on a trait of social anxiety might do so because he holds the view that the world is a harsh and competitive place in which he lacks the personal skills to compete (Schlenker and Leary 1982).

Although traits are generally regarded as an integral part of the self-system, some psychologists have argued that traits do not actually exist and that people's behaviour is simply an expression of socially determined responses to specific types of social situations (Mischel 1973). This idea has some intuitive appeal. For example, patients in hospital are expected to behave in ways that are quite different to doctors and nurses, suggesting that each group has a set of expectations about the *social role* that they must adopt in such settings. Similarly, when two friends enter a lift full of people, they typically stop talking to each other and avoid eye contact with others in the lift. Clearly, it would be a nonsense to suggest that they have a 'lift-trait', or that all nurses have a 'nurse-trait', and so on. So, Mischel's assertion that behaviours are determined by social roles, etiquettes and taboos has some validity. However, we would be most surprised to find a ward full of newly admitted patients all behaving in exactly the same way! In short, behaviour may be best viewed as an interaction between traits, situations and socially determined roles.

Self-schemas

According to some psychologists, self-relevant information about socially determined behaviour (such as nurse–patient roles) is held in cognitive units called *self-schemas* (Howard 1987; Mark *et al.* 1997). Self-schemas are hypothetical units of knowledge that contain highly organised information about aspects of the self. For example, individuals may have a self-schema for their body image, gender roles, for being a student, nurse, patient, father, son, mother, daughter, etc. A number of psychologists have taken this idea further by arguing that the apparent existence of self-schemas should lead us to think of *multiple selves* rather than a single self-concept that would lead to consistent behaviour across all situations (Gergen 1971; Markus and Sentis 1982; Markus and Nurius 1986). Rather, multiple selves might lead to variations in behaviour across situations, as determined by the *role expectations* inherent in any given aspect of self (you may find it easier to think of individuals donning different 'hats' depending upon the situations they find themselves in). For example, a business man may have a self-schema that involves acting with a measure of aggressiveness and competitiveness towards other male colleagues at work, whilst at home he may display kindness and gentleness towards his son, concordant with his self-schema for being a good father.

Occasionally, the roles inherent in these differing aspects of self may conflict and disrupt interpersonal relationships. This may occur when a student nurse's expectations, contained in her self-schema for being a good student, conflict with her partner's self-schema for what constitutes a good wife.

Self-esteem

Self-esteem, the fourth component of the self-system, has been tradition-ally defined as a global phenomenon, which is either high or low (Coopersmith 1967). More recently, however, Harter (1988a; 1988b) has suggested that self-esteem is composed of a number of components relating to important aspects of self that include dimensions such as scholastic competence, athletic ability, social acceptance, conduct of behaviour and physical appearance. According to Harter, it is possible to have low self-esteem on one, or more, of these components, whilst still feeling generally good about oneself. This idea, which is remi-niscent of the multiple selves concept, is relevant to our understanding of human behaviour. For example, a physically handicapped boy may experience a consistent drop in self-esteem whenever events cause him to focus on the physical limitations imposed on him by his disability, whilst still enjoying a globally high self-esteem, because he is academically able and popular with his peers.

Viewed from the latter perspective, we may conclude that individuals have a high self-esteem when, on balance, the things they like about themselves outweigh the things they do not like. This positive balance appears to be the norm and most people maintain a relatively high self-esteem throughout life (Harter 1985). Whilst this balance may be temporarily altered by transient life events, the indi-vidual's self-esteem normally returns quickly to its baseline. Of course, this is not always the case. Significant events, such as unemployment, physical and mental illness, can adversely affect the way the individual perceives him or herself, so that the balance of self-esteem is negatively altered over longer periods of time or, in some instances, permanently.

Transitional life stages, such as adolescence, parenthood and retirement, may exert a similarly negative effect on self-esteem (Simmons *et al.* 1983). Such events typically challenge the individual and can result in a loss of self-esteem when a) the individual doubts his or her ability to cope or b) when the individual's actual behaviour falls short of personal expectations, or those of others. For example, a student will experience a loss of self-esteem if she gets low marks in an exam that she has expected to do well in or if she tries hard to make herself attractive to someone who subsequently puts her down.

Rogers (1951) conceptualised this phenomenon as a basic mis-match between the individual's *ideal and actual self*, and proposed that chronic anxiety or depression may occur when individuals consistently set themselves ideals that they cannot hope to achieve. This notion has clinical utility outside psychiatry. For example, it is easy to envisage how a young, attractive female disfigured by burns could experience a marked and enduring loss of self-esteem, given that her ideal body image no longer matched reality. Similarly, Roger's framework would allow us to understand how a first-time mother could experience feelings of inadequacy, anger and depression, in struggling to cope with a baby that does not fit the norm or ideal portrayed in advertisements for baby products.

Whilst the balance of self-esteem can vary as a function of situational factors (as in the latter examples), many psychologists believe that the roots of a positive self-esteem are sown during the early years of life, when the child experiences unconditional love and nurturance. By the same token, adverse experiences during childhood can result in problems with self-esteem later in life. Buss (1980), for example, argues that a pattern of inconsistent parenting, negative feedback and emotional and physical abuse can result in chronic feelings of low self-worth. Indeed, it is not difficult to envisage why this may occur. The very young child has an under-developed concept of self that is being shaped by feedback from significant others. If that feedback is consistently negative or erratic, he or she is at risk of developing a deeply ingrained dislike of self and/or a strong sense of insecurity.

Bee (1997) argues that the development of chronic feelings of low self-worth during childhood hinders the establishment of normal social relationships, which in extreme cases may lead to the development of sociopathic and destructive behaviour in children and adults. Exactly why this should be is unclear, but Berkowitz (1993), an acknowledged expert on aggression, argues that most of us tend to be nasty to others when we feel bad about ourselves (you might like to check out this hypothesis the next time you have had a bad day). In the case of individuals with a chronically low self-esteem, it appears that an intense dislike of self is transferred into an intense dislike of others.

We will investigate the root causes of anger and aggression later in this text. For now, however, we have reached the point where it is possible to develop a simple model based on the premise that self-esteem is a function of an overall balance of positive and negative aspects of self (see Figure 2.2). According to this model, the balance is affected in varying degrees by the legacy of early childhood experiences, major and minor life events, transitional life stages and our expectations and achievements.

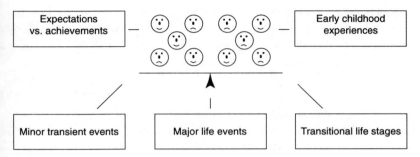

FIGURE 2.2 The components of self-esteem

The stability of the self-system

Once developed, the traits, belief systems and self-esteem that comprise the self-system remain relatively stable and change only gradually thoughout adult life (Woods and Britton 1985). This stability affords the individual a sense of continuity that is resistant to situational pressures and the effects of time.

This stability emerges quite clearly from research carried out on elderly populations. Elderly people typically report that they do not actually feel any different in psychological terms, and longitudinal studies confirm that their traits tend to alter very little over time (Birren and Schaie 1985). In fact, the only reliable change in personality demonstrated by researchers has consisted of a small shift towards conservatism and rigidity (Kermis 1984). If anything, this suggests that traits are likely to become even more fixed with the passing of time.

Changes in personality can occur as a consequence of illness, either through stress or direct cerebral damage in the cases of strokes or lesions. Notably, however, the occurrence of illness typically results in an exaggeration of existing traits, rather than the formation of new ones (Lancaster 1984). When the stability of the self-system does break down, it is invariably caused by significant life events or transitional life stages that have the effect of evoking a major reappraisal and reorganisation of the self. Perhaps the most notable of these transitional stages occurs during adolescence, when some individuals experience an 'identity crisis' that is linked to a difficulty in making the changes in self-concept necessary to view oneself as an adult (Marcia 1980). In some societies, specific rituals or 'rites of passage' help the individual to make this change. In the western world, however, it is often significant events, such as starting a full-time job or leaving home, that mark the change in the individual's status. This may explain why Waterman's (1985) research revealed that some teenagers experienced a crisis only after entering higher education or paid employment.

Erikson (1950) argued that adolescent crises are triggered when the teenager questions his or her own identity and has difficulty reconciling personal beliefs and values with those of significant others or society at large. Given this perspective, it is not difficult to envisage why other relatively common events, such as having an extra-marital affair or being sacked by one's employer, can cause self reappraisal, intra-personal conflict and much soul-searching. From this, we can deduce that personal crises are not evoked exclusively by major events like bereavement, acute illness or the threat of dying, and that disequilibrium may be evoked by any event that threatens the integrity of the self-system, be it seemingly big or small.

Summary

The self-system is composed of four basic components – body image, traits, belief systems and self-esteem – which can each exert a significant effect on how we perceive ourselves and others. This system is relatively robust and stable, evolving only gradually over time as a function of personal experiences, feedback from others and self-reappraisals.

Information about social roles and expectancies is contained in self-schemas, and the individual's behaviour may be influenced by the 'hat' they are wearing at any point in time.

Self-esteem fluctuates around a generally positive baseline as a function of minor hassles and uplifts. Occasionally, however, significant life events or transitional life stages may result in a major self-reappraisal and a shift in the balance of self-esteem, which may be enduring or permanent.

Chapter 3

The development of the self in childhood

Learning outcomes

By the end of this chapter you should be able to:

- Explain the importance of a secure emotional base in childhood.
- Describe how the self develops with special reference to cognitive self-awareness, social cognition and the social group.
- Outline how individual differences in self-awareness can affect behaviour.

The early years of life

During the early years of life, the developing child is faced with four major developmental tasks. It must develop *motor skills*, so that it is able to manipulate objects and move itself from a to b. The child must also develop *cognitively*, so that it can master language and communicate with others. It must develop *emotionally*, so that it can cope with its own emotions and adapt them to take account of others' needs, and it must develop *socially*, so that it can thrive within its social group.

The normal development of these skills is largely dependent upon the availability of a secure emotional base, such as is normally provided by the child's mother, father or guardian. When the child has a safe base, it is encouraged to explore the world and hone its motor and language skills; similarly, the child is most likely to develop healthy social relationships when it feels secure.

The development of a secure emotional base

The importance of a secure emotional base for normal personal and social development has been emphasised by a number of prominent theorists over the years, including Erikson, Bowlby and Ainsworth.

Erikson (1950), for example, argued that the child's experiences during the first year of life lead to the development of an enduring sense of *trust or mistrust* of others, which has a pervasive effect on the child's ability to build successful relationships. Bee (1997) states that research supports this view and points out that the children most at risk of developing abnormal social relationships are those exposed to harsh and erratic parenting during the early years of life.

The perceived importance of these relationships led to the development of *attachment theory* and the subsequent study of parent–child interactions by two prominent researchers, Bowlby (1969; 1975; 1980) and Ainsworth *et al.* (1978). According to attachment theory, the formation of close emotional bonds is necessary for successful child development and successful parenting. These bonds provide the child with a sense of security and confidence that facilitates the development of normal social relationships, and they provide the parents with a sense of intimacy that helps to cement a loving relationship with their child. Research has shown that children who lack these bonds carry a higher risk of abnormal social development, and parents who lack them are more likely to abuse their offspring (Sroufe 1989; Cohn 1990; Bee 1997).

According to Bowlby (1980, p. 39), attachment behaviours may be defined as 'any form of behaviour that results in a person attaining or retaining proximity to some differentiated and preferred person'. These special child–parent interactions can be easily recognised by the presence of reciprocal eye contact, verbalisations, laughing, play, touch and proximity seeking behaviours. Whilst the presence of such behaviours signals the development of a secure parent–child relationship (Bee 1997), their absence is normally regarded as a cause for some concern.

Parent–child attachments can become inhibited or blocked for reasons that are varied and complex. However, research has shown that problems frequently occur when:

1   the mother's own adverse childhood experiences result in negative self-expectations and a lack of confidence in the ability to be a good mother (Sroufe and Fleeson 1986);
2   the mother is suffering from a psychological disorder, such as post-natal depression, that renders her emotionally flat and distant from others (Field *et al.* 1990; Kendall-Tackett and Kaufman-Kantor 1993; Cox and Holden 1994).
3   the child has a congenital disability, such as blindness, that hinders the development of spontaneous attachment behaviours. (Fortunately, in such cases, the parents can be taught to respond successfully to touch and other cues as a medium for the development of a healthy bond [Fraiberg 1975].)

In addition, bonding may be impeded when the child is hospitalised in a neonatal intensive care unit as a result of premature delivery, genetic disorders or physical complications at birth (Hyland and Donaldson 1989). Under such circumstances, a number of factors may impede the process of bonding which include:

- Feeling that the staff 'own' the baby.
- Being put off by clinical apparatus, such as the incubator, feeding tubes and monitoring devices.
- Being worried about causing infection or harming the baby in some other way.
- Feeling disappointed by the absence of normal attachment cues emanating from the baby.
- Being put off by the physical unattractiveness of a very premature baby.
- Being in physical pain or discomfort as a result of a caesarean section, episiostomy, pre-eclampsia or other complications post-partum.
- Feeling guilty about the child's condition and/or being made to feel responsible because of judgemental staff attitudes.

Focus on clinical practice: children's reactions to separation

Behavioural and emotional effects of separation

Bowlby (1975; 1980) has argued that young children, separated from their parents in strange environments and cared for by a succession of strangers, often display a characteristic pattern of behaviour that consists of protest, despair and detachment.

According to Bowlby, *protest* consists of behaviours that include crying loudly, shaking the cot sides, throwing itself, or other objects, about and looking and listening eagerly for cues that might suggest the return of the attachment figure. He noted, too, that children placed in residential nursery care (i.e. because their mothers were hospitalised and unable to care for them) often showed a typical sequence of behaviours that included crying, clinging and screaming when the mothers had to leave, followed by a refusal to eat, get dressed and undressed, and to use the potty, etc.

Bowlby observed that this initial protest phase was often followed by a period of *despair*, manifested by an absence of overt, demonstrative behaviours and by emotional withdrawal. He argued that although the child's longing for the mother was not diminished, the hope that she would return had begun to fade.

He also noted that during prolonged periods of separation, the child entered a stage of apparent emotional *detachment* and exhibited normal behaviours that gave a false impression of recovery. Bowlby observed, however, that closer examination of the child's behaviour often provided evidence of continued stress. For example, one child was found repetitively muttering under his breath the words 'my mummy's coming soon . . . my mummy's coming soon' (Bowlby 1980, p. 11).

Perhaps the most surprising of Bowlby's findings, however, was the observation that children often ignored their mothers when reunited with them and, in some instances, displayed overt hostility towards them.

Understanding children's reactions to separation

Children often perceive the world in ways quite different to adults, and this may affect the way in which they subsequently respond to periods of separation. For example, Bibbace and Walsh (1980) found that young children often believe that being ill is a punishment for being bad or naughty, and as a consequence the child may feel that being hospitalised is yet a further punishment for some wrongdoing. Similarly, children have a different perception of time. Thus, a week may feel like a month and month like a year (Wilkinson 1988). Accordingly, reassurances that the separation period will be short may fall on deaf ears, and it is even conceivable the hospitalised child may feel deceived or rejected in some way. It is against this background that we must view the three primary emotional responses to separation: *anxiety*, *anger* and *sorrow*.

According to Bowlby, attachment behaviours are always goal driven or goal directed. Indeed, studies of primates and humans suggest that animals have a strong, intrinsic or biological drive to be close to the main attachment figure (which is often the mother). As a consequence, separation, or the threat of separation, typically results in anxiety which is commonly exacerbated by strange environments and the presence of strangers (Ainsworth 1982). The behaviours displayed during the protest phase may be viewed as attempts to gain the attention of the attachment figure in order to regain the safety that his or her close proximity offers. When such attempts fail, the response is often one of anger, which may be seen as a crude reflexive or instinctive emotion that occurs in response to frustration. In older children, however, anger may be a function of attributional processes. Weiner (1986), for example, has argued that anger often occurs when people view an untoward event as something that is intentional, malevolent and avoidable. Hence, it is conceivable that a child may hold the parent responsible for its separation, whilst not being quite old enough to understand that it is illness (or some other cause) that has necessitated separation, rather than some malevolent intent.

According to Bowlby, anger should be seen as a functional and natural response to separation, which normally wanes once the child is reunited with the parent. However, anger may be viewed as dysfunctional when it is frequent, uncontrolled and destructive, something that Bowlby claims is most likely to be observed in children frequently abandoned when young.

When neither protest nor anger results in reunion, the child may experience a sense of hopelessness and sorrow, which is caused by the loss of the valued bond with the primary attachment figure or figures (Brown 1982). Indeed, Bowlby's three phases of protest, despair and detachment bear much in common with the phenomenon now known as *learned helplessness*, which we will discuss in Part Two.

Individual differences in response to separation

Although attachment behaviours such as clinging and protesting can be seen in children of all ages, Ainsworth (1978) found that reliable individual differences in attachment behaviours may be witnessed in children from about 12 months of age. Her findings were based upon the extensive use of an experimental paradigm called the '*strange situation*', which was used to explore children's reactions to separation and reunion with their mothers. On the basis of many observations, Ainsworth noted that whilst some children unreservedly welcomed their mothers back following a brief period of separation in a strange and unfamiliar environment, others showed evidence of ambivalence and even anger, resistance and avoidant behaviours (such as gaze aversion) when reunited with their mothers. She concluded that such differences in behaviour were a function of the extent to which the child was *securely* or *insecurely attached* to the mother.

Whilst such individual differences in response may well be a function of the quality of the child–parent attachment, it is important to note that situational or environmental factors may also play a significant role in determining the child's response to enforced separation. For example, Main and Weston (1982) note that avoidance behaviour is commonly a function of the length and stressfullness of the separation. Similarly, it seems likely that the experience of separation due to illness will be influenced by the subsequent quality of nursing care and the nature of the environment in which the care takes place. Taking, for example, Bowlby's observation that separation anxiety is likely to occur when the child is cared for by a succession of strangers, it is not difficult to understand why primary nursing in a children's environment should always be preferred to task-oriented nursing, where patients are not allocated to specific care staff.

It is also likely that separation anxiety will be mediated by the parents' reactions, as they provide the child with powerful non-verbal cues that indicate the seriousness, or otherwise, of the situation. If the parents' facial expressions or tone of voice inform the child that the situation is serious, it is more likely to feel anxious, rejected and abandoned when the parents have to leave. Anxiety and despair may also be increased by procedures that limit physical contact and increase the child's sense of isolation (such as some forms of barrier nursing), and by situations where the child is unable to receive regular visits from the primary care givers.

Finally, individual differences in children make it difficult to generate precise guidelines about how long separation must occur before the child begins to feel distressed. However, as a general rule it is possible to state that young children are likely to be distressed by relatively short periods of separation (such as an overnight stay in hospital), whilst older children are more likely to be distressed by enforced periods of separation lasting days, weeks or longer (as might occur in institutional settings).

The emergence of cognitive self-awareness

During the first year of life, the child is preoccupied with honing the sensory-motor skills that allow it to touch, taste and explore its environment (Piaget 1954). During this stage of development, the child lives very much in the 'here and now' and there is little evidence that it actively plans, intends or reflects consciously on the consequences of its actions. Buss (1980) refers to this state of being as a *sensory awareness* of self and argues that it is very much on a par with the type of awareness that is found in cats and dogs.

During the second year of life, however, a marked change in the child's self-awareness becomes evident through its actions. At around the age of 2, for example, children begin to recognise themselves in the mirror, they begin to self-name in photographs, they become aware of their sexual identity, they become aware of their appearance and dress and they start to label toys and other personal possessions as 'my toy' etc. (Lewis and Brooks-Gunn 1979; Kagan 1982). It is also around this age that toddlers display the temper tantrums associated with the 'terrible twos', and, as many parents will bear witness to, children often display such behaviours in the realisation that they can exert a strong influence on the parents' subsequent behaviour.

Taken together, these phenomena suggest that the child is becoming aware of itself as a unique, social individual, which Buss (1980) suggests reflects the emergence of a *cognitive self-awareness* that may be defined as the ability to be an object of one's own knowledge and to reflect on who and what we are. This capability appears to represent a qualitative change in cognitive functions that facilitate the development of the social self.

Cognitive development, social cognition and the self-system

How humans develop into sophisticated social beings is a complex puzzle, and our task is not to dwell on the topic in depth. However, a number of things occur around the second year of life that might feasibly combine to facilitate cognitive self-awareness. First, there is a three- to fourfold increase in the size of the cortex and myelinisation of neural pathways occurring between birth and 2 to 3 years of age (Nowakowski 1987). Second, the brain's capacity to process, store and recall information is greatly increased (Bee 1997); and third, the child begins to master language, which gives it the ability to conceptualise events and emotions and to communicate with itself and others (Bates *et al.* 1987). Taken together, it seems likely that these developments allow the child to reflect on the causes and consequences of its actions, to perceive the world from others' perspectives and to share their perceptions, opinions, values and beliefs.

These reflective thoughts are sometimes collectively labelled *social cognition*, which may be broadly defined as the understanding of self and others that results from self-reflection in the context of social interaction. Such processes appear to be very important, as it is argued that the child comes to know itself by reflecting on the feedback provided by others, and comes to understand others' motives and feelings by reflecting on the consequences of its own behaviour (Cooley

1902; Mead 1934; Hastrup 1995). Although this may sound complex, it is easy to relate to at a personal level. For example, you would probably reflect on your actions if a close friend told you that you were basically self-centred and egotistical, and similarly you would, no doubt, be concerned if your actions caused someone else acute embarrassment.

Without social cognition, it seems likely that the child would be unable to understand itself or others and would remain an outcast, unable to learn the implicit rules that govern social behaviour. It is noteworthy that this deficit is a core feature of childhood *autism* (Hobson 1993).

The role of the social group in self-development

Some psychologists have argued that the self-system has evolved out of the need to regulate and modify personal behaviour within the social groups we inhabit (Trower *et al.* 1990). In doing so, we look to others to obtain information about the type of person we are and we look for information that tells us whether or not our behaviour (or our appearance) is socially acceptable (Cooley 1902; Mead 1934; Sullivan 1953; Goffman 1959; Argyle 1983). Furthermore, Bandura (1986) has argued that we model our behaviour on significant others within our social group, whilst Bee (1997) states that their standards help shape our own personal beliefs and values. This perspective is supported by a) *social comparison theory*, which proposes that we are *driven* to compare ourselves with others (Festinger 1954; Bem 1972) and b) research emanating from developmental psychology, which shows that self-comparison with others is an integral part of self-development.

These comparative processes show a clear developmental trend. That is, between the ages of about 2 and 6, children's self-comparisons are based upon external, physical features and abilities (such as how tall, small, fast or slow they are in relation to others), whereas from the age of about 7 or 8, children start to make more sophisticated comparisons based upon internal, psychological attributes (such as how clever, stupid, outgoing or introverted they are in relation to others) (Montemayor and Eisen 1977; Ruble 1987).

James (1995) argues that our concept of self develops out of self–other comparisons, and according to social comparison theory, we typically make such comparisons with others similar in appearance, intellect, social class, etc., presumably because they are unlikely to make us feel uncomfortable or inferior (Bem 1972). However, research shows that pre-school children, and those up to the age of about 6, tend to make comparisons with dissimilar others, such as parents and older siblings. By the time they reach secondary school, however, the importance of being like others in the social group reaches a peak (Sulls and Mullen 1982). Whilst this may result in financial pressures on parents to buy the latest designer jeans or trainers, it can also result in self-consciousness and a significant loss of self-esteem (James 1995) for children who are 'different', because they are overly tall, small, thin or fat, early or late entering puberty, etc., or for those who have some physical or psychological handicap.

Whilst the social group undoubtedly plays an important role in shaping the way in which we develop, it is evident that individuals sometimes develop in ways that are in direct conflict with significant others, such as family or even society at large. This suggests that both internal and external forces are important in shaping the self. Indeed, Maslow (1970) suggested that we have a strong internal drive to meet our own intrinsic goals and aspirations. Furthermore, we tend to become less reliant on comparisons with others for a feeling of self-worth or esteem as we age (Kimmel 1990), although, as we will see next, there is evidence that some adults continue to be highly reliant on others to maintain a positive self-image.

Individuals' differences in self-awareness

So far we have learnt that small children are particularly reliant on feedback from others to build a picture or model of themselves, but let us turn our discussion back to adults for a moment. Ask yourself, how reliant are you on others to provide positive feedback about your achievements and how important are their reactions for your self-esteem? You might find that this is partly dependent upon the situation you find yourself in. For example, you might recall having felt a greater need for positive feedback and reassurance when you found yourself in a novel or unfamiliar situation that made you insecure. Similarly, we might well imagine that an elderly woman rendered incontinent and immobile by a stroke would seek extra reassurance from family or nurses that she was still worthy of respect and attention.

In such circumstances, we are likely to pay particular attention to others' reactions to us. However, some psychologists have found that there are significant variations in the extent to which individuals are habitually reliant on feedback from others for checking the appropriateness of their behaviour or their self-worth. These differences are deemed to be due to trait-like dispositions that lead some individuals to be more self-conscious or self-aware than others (Snyder 1974; Fenigstein *et al.* 1975). For example, individuals high in the trait of *public self-consciousness* (PUBSC) are particularly concerned to present a favourable public image and closely monitor others' reactions towards them. Conversely, individuals high in private self-consciousness (PVSC) are less aware and concerned about others' reactions towards them and, as a consequence, are less likely to conform to group pressure when it involves conflict with their own personal beliefs or values (Fenigstein 1979)).

What causes PUBSC is unclear, although it is known that people who are high in this trait are more likely to experience social anxiety and embarrassment and are more likely to have a low self-esteem (Buss 1980; Cheek and Melchoir 1990). Perhaps, then, such individuals actively pay special attention to others' reactions because of a strong need to seek their reassurance. Whilst this type of behaviour may well be a function of personality traits, it is not difficult to envisage that PUBSC could also be induced by any public event that results in the individual being unsure about his or her ability to perform adequately (such as may occur when the student reluctantly gives a presentation to his or her peers).

Summary

The development of the self in childhood is facilitated by a secure emotional base and the growth of a close emotional bond with significant others, such as the child's parents or guardians. A sense of security gives the child confidence to explore its physical and social boundaries and underpins the development of normal social relationships with others. The feedback that the child receives from significant others provides important information about the self, in that the child who is loved comes to see itself as worthy of love and so develops a positive self-concept. By the reverse token, the child who receives erratic or consistently negative feedback from others is more likely to develop a negative self-concept and to have difficulty establishing and maintaining intimate relationships with others.

During the first year of life, the child's sense of self is limited to a basic form of sensory self-awareness that precludes conscious and deliberative self-reflection. From the second year of life onwards, however, the child becomes aware of itself as a social object and is gradually able to reflect with increasing sophistication upon its internal and external attributes and the causes and consequences of its own, and others', behaviour.

This qualitative change in cognitive ability is probably a function of increased brain capacity that is associated with the development of language and changes in the power of memory. The emergence of cognitive self-awareness heralds the development of the social self, and the beliefs, opinions and attitudes of significant others are gradually transfused into core, internal, self-standards that shape the individual's general behaviour and sense of self. In short, cognitive and emotional factors both play a crucial role in moulding the self. Cognitive self-awareness facilitates the development of social cognition and self-reflection, and a secure emotional base provides a platform for the development of normal social relationships with others.

Individuals differ in the extent to which they are self-aware or self-conscious. Individuals high in public self-consciousness, for example, are keenly aware of themselves as social objects and are particularly attentive to others' reactions towards them. Although public and private self-consciousness are treated as traits, any event or situation that draws adverse or unwanted attention to self-appearance or performance is highly likely to elicit acute public self-consciousness in all or most individuals. Finally, it is worth noting that the trait of public self-consciousness, and the self–other monitoring and checking that stems from it, has been linked to low self-esteem and a negative self-concept.

Chapter 4

Evaluating and protecting the self

Learning outcomes

By the end of this chapter you should be able to:

- Describe the five self-evaluative emotions.
- Outline the function of defence mechanisms, such as denial, downward social comparison and self-handicapping.
- Explain the difference between denial and self-illusory perceptions.

The self-evaluative emotions

So far we have learnt that others play a crucial role in the development of the self-system and that we continue to make self-comparisons with others throughout adult life, not least as a means of checking the appropriateness of our behaviour. Although most people do not feel continually anxious, events do occasionally occur that cause us to feel unsure of our abilities. This often results in anxiety, awkwardness and an increase in self-awareness. These feelings typically arise out of a *fear of negative evaluation*, or negative self-comparisons with others, and a variety of terms such as embarrassment, self-consciousness, social anxiety, shame and guilt have been used to explain them.

In the following discussion, we will learn that each emotional state has a special relevance to clinical practice, regardless of whether the patient population is drawn from the very young or the very old, the physically frail or handicapped or the psychologically disturbed. Before we move on, however, I would like to point out that one could develop a strong case for examining the emotions associated with positive self-evaluation. Unfortunately, little research exists to support their study, primarily because psychologists have been concerned only with the negative effects of self-comparative processes. Despite this, you might find it of interest and value to reflect on how patients deal positively with adverse events that might otherwise cause them to be concerned about others' negative evaluation.

Self-consciousness

Self-consciousness is an experience that is characterised by uncomfortable feelings of acute self-awareness and anxiety that can occur when people believe that they are (or may be) judged negatively by others. Relatively little research has been carried out into the situational factors that can cause self-consciousness, but in carrying out some recent research, I ascertained that the following key factors are involved:

- A fear of negative evaluation.
- Novel situations and the presence of strangers.
- Situations where the individual feels conspicuous and the centre of others' unwanted attentions.
- Concerns about personal appearance.
- Being asked to do things in public that are normally socially taboo.

If you stop to consider these criteria in light of the types of situation that patients can find themselves in, it is not difficult to envisage why they sometimes feel self-conscious. Health professionals often ask patients to do things that involve forms of public self-exposure that would normally be socially unacceptable. Furthermore, negative changes in body image can evoke a heightened awareness of self, feelings of embarrassment and a fear of negative evaluation. To take a case in point, one woman in my study reported feeling acutely self-conscious when asked to show her unusual form of breast cancer to a large group of medical students (Russell 1996).

Whilst such events are undoubtedly traumatic, it is just as important to remember that 'routine' events, such as using a bedpan, being incontinent or being asked to remove your clothes, can also cause acute self-consciousness.

Social anxiety

Social anxiety is closely associated with self-consciousness and occurs when the individual is motivated to present a favourable public image, but doubts their ability to do so (Schlenker and Leary 1982). Social anxiety is characterised by a fear of negative evaluation that is frequently combined with social avoidance of activities that might lead to public ridicule (Watson and Friend 1969).

Social anxiety is relatively commonplace and is usually situationally induced and transient. However, it may occasionally take the form of crippling, trait-like doubts that lead to avoidance of social situations. Chronic social anxiety may be linked to deeply ingrained doubts about one's ability to function competently in the public domain (Buss 1980; Beck and Emery 1985), but it may also be induced by any illness, trauma or clinical procedure that the patient believes will result in subsequent public censure or ridicule.

Although social anxiety is typically viewed as a psychiatric or mental health problem, it is easy to envisage why an individual with a stammer or a patient left with slurred speech following a stroke, might become extremely anxious at the prospect of any public activity. Indeed, social anxiety may be found in any client or patient population.

Embarrassment and shame

Embarrassment occurs when the individual transgresses some social rule, boundary, etiquette or taboo, and there is some overlap with self-consciousness. However, embarrassment and self-consciousness are usually treated as two distinct constructs, because embarrassment is generally regarded as less traumatic than self-consciousness and because it is possible to be embarrassed on someone else's behalf without feeling self-conscious yourself. This is termed vicarious embarrassment (Edelman 1981).

Harré (1990) argues that embarrassment functions as a largely non-verbal, social signal that is sent by the transgressor and received automatically by a recipient audience. Behaviours, such as blushing, eye gaze directed at the floor and fidgeting, indicate to the audience that the transgressor is aware of his or her 'error', which allows the audience the option of ignoring the error or providing reassurance that all is well. Harré argues that we learn to detect these cues and respond to them in such a way that it becomes an automatic and involuntary process. (Which might explain why we cannot help feeling embarrassed about the antics of purely fictional characters, such as Dell Boy in *Only Fools and Horses* and Basil Fawlty in *Fawlty Towers*). There is a serious side to this, of course. Feeling embarrassed is unpleasant and there is a danger that the types of event that can lead to its occurrence in clinical settings become regarded as so common and trivial by staff, that their significance is overlooked. For this reason, it is important occasionally to put yourself in the 'patient's shoes', in addition to being alert to non-verbal cues that may indicate that the patient feels awkward and uncomfortable.

Embarrassment and shame are interrelated in that they both occur when there is some transgression of social rules or etiquette (Buss 1980; Edelman 1981). However, whereas embarrassment is generally regarded as a transient state, associated with minor transgressions of social rules and etiquettes, shame is perceived as an enduring state, which is linked to more serious transgressions that are suggestive of some gross personal inadequacy or immoral act (Castalfranchi and Poggi 1990; Gibbons 1990). To take an example, a man might feel too embarrassed to admit to casualty staff that his wife had given him a black eye, whilst he might be too ashamed to admit that it had occurred as he was beating her up.

Bradbury (1993) argues that facially disfigured individuals sometimes experience shame, because people hold the deeply entrenched belief that good is beautiful and ugly is evil and immoral (if you doubt this, spend an evening watching the ways in which heroes and villains are differentially portrayed in films, advertisements and even fairy tales!). Furthermore, disfigured people are sometimes held responsible for their condition, on the basis that they *could* seek corrective plastic surgery if they so wished.

It is important to note that negative staff attitudes may reinforce (if not cause) shame in vulnerable patients. Stockwell (1984), for example, found that general nursing staff often held negative and judgemental attitudes towards certain categories of patient, such as homosexuals, psychiatric patients and those who were admitted following an overdose attempt. This is bad practice and we can state that whenever staff adopt a position that purports to give them the higher moral ground, the patient is likely to respond with a sense of inferiority and shame or, alternatively, anger and hostility.

Guilt

Guilt and shame are similar emotional states in that they both result from a transgression of moral standards, emanating from the individual, an organisation or society at large. However, Higgins (1990) argues that guilt and shame are readily distinguishable, because guilt is experienced only when the transgressor believes that his or her actions have resulted in harm to others. Take, for example, an adult woman who has unsuccessfully attempted to commit suicide. She may feel ashamed about having attempted suicide, but she will only feel guilty if she perceives that her actions have caused others, such as her family, distress. Of course, she could also feel guilty about failing to kill herself, particularly if she believed that success would have relieved them of her burden.

As we will see later, guilt is often prominent in depression and in bereavement reactions and is, therefore, likely to be frequently witnessed by nurses across a wide variety of clinical settings.

Summary so far

So far we have discussed five emotions or states that each result from actual or anticipatory negative self-evaluation (see Figure 4.1). Social anxiety typically results in anticipation of a negative event, self-consciousness and embarrassment often arise during an ongoing event, and guilt and shame are emotional states that occur in response to failure. At the core of each is a heightened sense of self that is accompanied by feelings that are distinctly unpleasant. Many types of event can give rise to these states and they may be found in all areas of clinical practice, regardless of whether one is dealing with children or adults or individuals with physical or psychological problems.

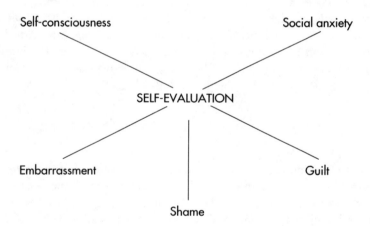

FIGURE 4.1 The five self-evaluative emotions

Protecting the self

Theorists have long been fascinated by the mechanisms used by individuals to protect their self-concept. During the early part of this century, prominent psychiatrists, such as Freud (1901), proposed that people use *mental defence mechanisms* to protect themselves from feelings of overwhelming anxiety, guilt and shame. These mechanisms were assumed to be employed unconsciously, and their presence (when observed via the patient's abnormal behaviour) was taken as evidence of some repressed intra-personal conflict that stemmed from instinctual urges to commit acts that were socially unacceptable. Although the theoretical assumptions that underpin the Freudian or psychoanalytic perspective have fallen out of favour in mainstream psychology, many of the concepts are still widely applied in clinical practice. For example, the defence mechanism of *denial* is commonly used to describe the individual's initial response to traumatic, personal events. The term *projection* is used to describe the anger and aggression that may result when an individual unconsciously shifts feelings of self-blame and guilt onto an innocent third party (often the hapless nurse or doctor), and the term *sublimation* is used to describe the channelling of socially unacceptable impulses into socially acceptable outlets as, for example, may occur when feelings of aggression are vented legally during a game such as football.

More recently, social psychologists have begun to use alternative theoretical perspectives to investigate how people defend the self when it is threatened by major events, such as cancer, heart disease, disfigurement and even death (Lazarus 1983; Taylor and Brown 1988), and their efforts have largely focused on the adaptive role of *illusory self-perceptions* in maintaining a high self-esteem and sense of personal control.

The theoretical frameworks that underpin the psychoanalytic and social-psychological fields of research are fundamentally different and their detailed discussion is beyond the scope of this text. However, there are two relevant points that we can usefully extract: first, they both hold the common position that defence mechanisms protect the individual from threats that might otherwise disrupt or destroy the integrity of the self-system; and second, they differ in that psychiatry has typically viewed these mechanisms as maladaptive, abnormal and undesirable, whilst social psychologists have broadly perceived them as adaptive and normal. Whilst both positions arguably have some merit, we will adopt the following working definition:

> Individuals employ a range of defensive strategies when the integrity of the self-system is threatened. These strategies or

mechanisms are often automatically employed and individuals may be unaware that they are using them. As their function is to protect the self, they should be treated as adaptive unless they start to interfere with normal social functioning in a self-destructive or anti-social way.

Before we take this discussion any further, I would like to offer you a case study that graphically illustrates how reality may be distorted to protect the self. The individual concerned was a smart, though sombrely dressed, single man in his fifties who suffered from recurrent bouts of moderate to severe depression. He always carried a black attaché case that was filled with 'personal correspondence with the queen', which he claimed dated back many years. In his letters he had offered the queen 'advice and guidance' that he truly believed to be well received. However, clinical staff knew that, although he had written regularly to the queen, he had only ever received polite replies from anonymous civil servants at the palace.

So why did he persist with the charade? Well, he was a very lonely man, with no job and no friends to boost his self-esteem. The letters he carried appeared to be part of a delusional belief system that provided him with a sense of importance that was vital to his well-being. In short, his self-delusions were adaptive and there was general agreement amongst the staff that we should not seek to challenge them, without first devising some alternative way of maintaining a positive self-esteem. This latter point is important, regardless of whether a patient is distorting reality to deal with loneliness and a low self-esteem, or is distorting reality due to a fear of dying from cancer.

Illusory self-perceptions

Although the latter scenario paints a picture of extremes – the social misfit who creates a delusional system in order to make himself feel important – you might be surprised to learn that social psychologists are uncovering evidence that suggests that we *all* distort reality in varying degrees in order to make ourselves feel good. Taylor and Brown (1988) label these distortions *illusory self-perceptions*, and state that a considerable body of research points to the fact that 'exaggerated perceptions of control or mastery, and unrealistic optimism are characteristic of human thought' (p. 193).

These illusory self-perceptions are bolstered by a range of *pre-conscious biases* that affect the way in which we process information available to us. For example, we tend to make internal attributions for successes (that is, attribute the cause of success to ourselves), whilst we tend to make external attributions for failures (that is, attribute the failure to others or other things) (Zuckerman 1979; Lewinsohn and Mischel 1980). This so-called *self-serving bias* is quite common and can be seen operating when a student blames the lecturer for failure to pass an assessment rather than her own lack of work during the year. Similarly, Silverman (1964) has found that we tend to recall successes more easily than failures, and Fiske and Taylor (1984) and Janis and Mann (1979) have shown that our prior expectations bias our judgements and cause us to gather and interpret information in such a way that our existing beliefs are upheld.

Taylor (1983) points out that cancer patients and their relatives often employ illusory self-perceptions in an effort to cope with potentially devastating situations. For example, Taylor found that cancer patients often showed a level of hope that was not supported by the 'facts', and noted that the optimism generated by this helped to create feelings of personal control and helped ward off a sense of hopelessness. Viewed from this perspective, it seems evident that seeing the world though rose-tinted glasses can be beneficial to our well-being, rather than detrimental.

Denial

Denial may be defined as a distortion or repudiation of reality, and it shares this core feature with illusory self-perceptions. In fact, the main feature distinguishing these two constructs is not a matter of the degree to which reality is distorted, but appears to rest on the fact that, historically, psychiatrists have generally perceived denial as maladaptive, whilst social psychologists have tended to view illusory self-perceptions as adaptive (Russell 1993). To avoid further conceptual confusion, we will simply adopt the position that denial is one of a range of illusory self-perceptions that should be regarded as adaptive unless its use starts to interfere with normal social functioning in an undesirable way.

Denial may be commonly observed in all areas of clinical practice, and leading researchers such as Lazarus (1983) have suggested that the ability to distort or negate the full impact of negative or disruptive change is an essential, adaptive coping response. This view is also mirrored in more recent research. For example, high levels of denial have been shown to facilitate recovery in the initial period following myocardial infarction and coronary bypass surgery (Levine *et al.* 1987; Folks *et al.* 1988), though there is a suggestion that the longer-term use of denial may adversely affect recovery from physical conditions (possibly because it may lead to non-compliance with medical advice).

Downward social comparison

Downward social comparison occurs when individuals make self-comparisons with others worse off than they are, as a means of reducing the magnitude of threat posed to the self (Wills 1982). This defence mechanism is commonly seen in individuals who are trying to cope with major life events, such as illness, and it is an adaptive, though arguably self-illusory, coping mechanism (Feldman 1995). For example, a mother who has a baby in neonatal intensive care, as a result of a pre-term delivery and hypoglycaemia, may lessen her anxiety by consoling herself that she is not as badly off as the mother whose child is being ventilated because of pneumonia and a collapsed lung.

Self-handicapping

Self-handicapping is a defence mechanism that involves attributing failure to some external cause (Jones and Pittman 1982). Like most defence mechanisms, its purpose is to negate threats to the self and boost self-esteem. However, self-handicapping can become a mal-adaptive response, when the triggering fear of failure is reinforced by the self-handicapping tactic. For example, a man may get drunk prior to an exam as a strategy that conveniently allows him to blame failure on the resulting hangover. Whilst this unconsciously motivated strategy may well suffice as a 'one-off' way of saving face, it would become mal-adaptive and self-destructive if he subsequently came to rely on alcohol *whenever* he was faced with a potentially evaluative social situation that carried the risk of failure.

Sadder but wiser? Self-focused attention and illusory self-perceptions

The final issue we will deal with in this first section concerns the effects of self-focused attention on self-esteem. In brief, you might imagine that by regularly focusing on your thoughts, feelings and motives you would learn more about yourself and eventually end up a happier person. However, you could be wrong. There is a strong body of evidence that shows that self-focused attention frequently results in a *lowering* of self-esteem (Duval and Wicklund 1972; Farber 1989; Gibbons 1990; Ingram 1990).

What can we make of this? Well, one way of viewing the evidence is to take the perspective that we defend our self-image by gently distorting reality (the illusory self-perception view) and ignoring unpalatable facts about ourselves that are revealed only by close self-scrutiny. We might also support this theoretically by using Rogers' (1951) ideal–actual-self model and hypothesising that focusing on the self leads to an awareness of discrepancies between what we think we are and what we actually are.

Indeed, Duval and Wicklund (1972) found experimental evidence to support just such a hypothesis, and a further piece of intriguing research, carried out by Alloy and Abramson in 1979, lent further weight to the argument. The latter investigators found that clinically depressed people were much more accurate in their self-appraisals than non-depressed people, leading to the suggestion that they were depressed because they knew more about themselves.

Many people, psychologists included, object to the idea that knowing yourself better should make you unhappier. Furthermore, the proposition flies in the face of the rationale behind interventions, such as psychotherapy, that are designed to make the individual happier through enhanced self-awareness. So, without being too controversial, let us extract one key point: it seems that focusing on the self *can* sometimes lead to a lowering of self-esteem. Now take this point and relate it to your own experiences. Ask yourself how frequently you focus on yourself and whether you are most likely to do so when something adverse occurs (like personal criticism from a close friend). Finally, ask yourself whether you think that events, such as surgery or mental illness, might lead patients to focus more closely on certain aspects of self, and reflect on what effect this might feasibly have.

Summary

So far we have learnt that the self-system is a complex psychological phenomenon that provides a window through which individuals view themselves and the world around them. The system plays a central role in determining how we perceive ourselves and others. If we are high in self-esteem, we tend to perceive others positively; if we are low in self-esteem, we tend to feel bad about ourselves and have difficulty with inter-personal relationships.

We are not born with a concept of self. It evolves gradually over time and is heavily influenced by the reactions of significant others as we compare and contrast our personal attributes, beliefs and behaviours. These self-evaluative processes, or social cognitions, can lead to a variety of emotional states such as self-consciousness, embarrassment, guilt and shame, and these all share the common characteristic that they involve uncomfortable feelings of self-awareness that result from actual or anticipatory negative evaluation. There are individual differences in the extent to which we continue to rely on others' feedback for our self-worth, but there are very few individuals who are totally uncaring about what others think of them.

Routine clinical tasks can subject the individual to various forms of public self-exposure that would normally be socially unacceptable, and these are likely to evoke self-consciousness and embarrassment. Negative and judgemental staff attitudes may heighten, or cause, a sense of shame in vulnerable patients, and guilt is likely to occur when the patient (or nurse) believes that his or her actions have resulted in harm to a third party.

When the self is threatened, we seek to defend our self-image by employing defensive strategies or illusory self-perceptions that bend or distort reality in varying degrees. These strategies are commonplace and generally adaptive and are particularly likely to be observed in clinical practice, where they are used to reduce feelings of anxiety and vulnerability that arise from physical or psychological threats to the individual's well-being.

MINI SELF-TEST

1   Briefly outline the main components of the self-system.

2   Describe what is meant by a self-schema.

3 List the phenomena that are likely to cause a drop in self-esteem.

4 Briefly outline social comparison theory and explain why we prefer to make comparisons with similar others.

5 Briefly explain how we come to acquire our internal self-standards.

6 Why is the development of a secure emotional base important for the development of healthy social relationships?

7 Describe the features of public self-consciousness.

8 Briefly compare and contrast each of the self-evaluative emotions.

9 Briefly explain the principal benefits derived from the use of strategies such as downward social comparison and self-handicapping.

10 What is the difference between illusory self-perceptions and denial, and when does their use become maladaptive?

REFLECTIVE SCENARIOS

Susan

Susan is eighteen months into her nursing course. She is very keen to do well, but her studies are being compromised by her partner's constant bickering when she comes home from work. He appears resentful of her work and her studying at home and she feels both guilty and resentful. *Explain what might be happening to their relationship with reference to concepts such as self-schemas, role expectations and multiple selves.*

Omar

Omar is 2½ years old and attends nursery full-time while his parents are at work. When he is collected in the evening, he typically responds by avoiding eye contact with them and ignoring all attempts to communicate. When they arrive home, he often flings a temper tantrum and occasionally bites and scratches anyone who attempts to console him. *How might we explain Omar's behaviour with reference to attachment theory and children's reactions to separation?*

Sarah

Sarah recently gave birth to a baby boy who was born prematurely at thirty-three weeks by emergency caesarean section. He has been nursed in neonatal intensive care for the past ten days due to physical complications. Although she is greatly concerned for his well-being, she cannot understand why she feels so distant from him.

Discuss the factors that might impede bonding with her child.

Matthew

Matthew is a 13-year-old boy with Downs Syndrome who has recently started at the local comprehensive after completing an extra year at primary school. He is generally regarded as enthusiastic and reasonably bright, although his IQ lies some way below average. Physically he is quite fit, but he has nystagmus and suffers from asthma, which is controlled by the use of inhalers. Although Matthew had few problems at his primary school, he was decidedly 'put out' at having to stay behind for a year and has been unable to re-establish the relationships that he had with his former friends. His teacher is concerned that he is not gelling with the class, and his parents are worried because he no longer wants to walk home from school and prefers, uncharacteristically, to stay in his room during the evening.

Discuss the possible causes of Matthew's behaviour with reference to social comparison theory, self-esteem and the self-evaluative emotions.

Panna

Panna is in her mid-fifties and was recently admitted to the Regional Burns and Plastic Surgery Unit with severe burns to her face, chest and abdomen. Although the medical staff are confident that she will survive, they anticipate that she will have problems adjusting to the prospect of corrective surgery and permanent scarring.

Using your knowledge of concepts such as ideal–actual self, stability of the self-system, social comparison theory and self-consciousness, discuss what effect the event is likely to have on her.

Robert

Robert is a 28-year-old man who has recently been promoted to the post of nurse-manager. Although he was initially pleased about his promotion, he harboured some doubts about his ability to do the job. Of late he has become very anxious when asked to speak in public or give presentations to his colleagues. In fact, on one day last week, he felt so bad that he phoned in sick.

Discuss Robert's behaviour with reference to social anxiety.

Liv and Karsten

Liv and Karsten have been happily married for more than forty years. However, Karsten has recently undergone a succession of treatments for cancer of the bowel that have been unsuccessful and he is now receiving palliative care at home. Although Karsten's prognosis is extremely poor, they both behave as though everything is more or less normal. This concerns the visiting district nurse who fears that Liv is going to come down with a hard bump when Karsten eventually passes away.

Discuss the extent to which the district nurse's fears are justified with reference to illusory self-perceptions and denial.

Suggested reading

Bee, H. (1997). *The Developing Child*. 8th ed. New York: HarperCollins.
This is a comprehensive book that should be of interest to any nurse working with children. Bee's style is authoritative but straightforward, and she never gets bogged down in irrelevant detail.

Buss, A. H. (1980). *Self-consciousness and Social Anxiety*. New York: W. H. Freeman and Co.
Although a little dated, this is probably still the best introductory text for anyone wanting to learn about the social evaluative emotions.

Feldman, R. S. (1995). *Social Psychology*. Chapters 4 and 5. The self: perceiving and understanding ourselves and well-being and health psychology. Englewood Cliffs, NJ: Prentice Hall.
This text provides a straightforward and well-written overview of how the self affects behaviour and health, viewed from social psychology. It also covers other potentially relevant theories and concepts that are beyond the scope of this text.

Lansdown, R., Rumsey, N., Bradbury, E., Carr, T. and Partridge, J. (1997). *Visibly Different: Coping with disfigurement*. Oxford: Butterworth Heinemann.
This is a well-written book about disfigurement aimed at both an academic and a public audience. It contains up-to-date research and contributions from individuals who are themselves disfigured.

Taylor, S. E. (1983). Adjustment to threatening events: A theory of cognitive adaptation. *American Psychologist* 38, 1161–1173.
This lucid paper provides an overview of the importance of mastery and control in adverse situations and it illustrates how illusory self-perception can protect the integrity of the self-system.

Part two

Reactions to change, challenging events and loss

Chapter 5

Stress, appraisal and coping

Learning outcomes

By the end of this chapter you should be able to:

- Describe the concepts of stress and threat appraisal.
- Describe the major factors that have been shown to mediate reactions to challenging or threatening events.
- Outline how an acute health crisis may develop.

The nature of stress

There can be few people in the western world who have not heard of stress, or who have not occasionally described their day to a colleague or friend as 'stressful'. Furthermore, stress cannot be dismissed as an irrelevant and minor side-effect of modern life, because, as we will learn in Part Four of this text, it has been linked to the onset of major disease and an overall increase in morbidity and mortality in vulnerable patients. Our first task, however, is to examine the basic nature of stress, so that we have a platform for discussion.

Stress is often conceptualised as comprising two basic dimensions: a *stressor*, such as the onset of illness or the threat posed to self-esteem by redundancy or exam failure, and a *stress response*, such as the feelings of tension and anxiety that may be experienced and the often invisible strain that is placed on the body's systems when the stress response is prolonged (Sarrafino 1994) (basic details of the physiological stress or 'alarm' response are given in Part four). In addition, a third dimension emerges from the *transactional view*, which depicts stress as a *process* involving an interaction between the challenging event, the subsequent threat perception and the coping responses available to the individual (Cox 1978; Lazarus and Folkman 1984). Viewed from this perspective, challenging events result in stress only when there is a *discrepancy* between the *demands* of the situation and the *resources* available to the individual. This is an important point. Significant events, such as hospitalisation, may result in initial anxiety for most patients, but if the patient views the reasons for admission as serious and beyond his or her control, stress is highly likely to result.

Life events

During the 1970s, psychologists were keen to establish what types of event might cause stress. This was accomplished by asking large, *normative populations* to rate the stressfulness of common events (Rahe and Arthur 1978). Not surprisingly, this research showed that people rated the death of a spouse or child as the most stressful, commonly occurring life event, followed by events such as severe illness, redundancy, divorce, etc. However, subsequent research questioned the value of such scales, on the basis that they provided little information about the response that could be expected at the *level of the individual* (Sarrafino 1994). We can relate this back to the transactional model, because life events result in stress only when individuals believe that the demands or challenges inherent in the situation will exceed their ability to cope. In short, not all events are *perceived as threatening*. Redundancy or divorce, for example, might come as a blessing in disguise. Similarly, events that would be rated as low in stress by the majority of people would be rated as highly stressful by a small, but significant, minority of individuals. For example, Christmas might be rated as highly stressful by someone who feels that the festive season only serves to remind them of their isolation from the rest of society; likewise a change in eating habits would be rated as stressful by someone suffering from anorexia nervosa.

Threat appraisal

Underpinning the transactional model is the assumption that, when faced with a challenging event, people try to ascertain whether the event poses a threat to their physical or psychological well-being and then make a judgement about how serious the threat may be (Cohen and Lazarus 1983). This cognitive assessment is termed the *primary* (or initial) *appraisal*, and if the event is perceived as threatening, a *secondary appraisal* is made, wherein the individual tries to assess whether or not they will be able to deal with the challenge successfully. In carrying out this appraisal, individuals may consider:

- Whether they have successfully dealt with similar events before.
- What resources they may draw on to help them deal with the event.
- How confident they feel about the likelihood of a successful outcome.

If the individual concludes that the event can be dealt with successfully, the threat is diminished and attention is diverted to other tasks.

However, if individuals conclude that they have no adequate way of dealing with the threat, they start to experience feelings of anxiety as the stress response is evoked.

Causes of stress

Whilst life event scales are not a wholly reliable indicator of stress at the level of the individual, it is possible to identify a number of general, or non-situation specific, factors that are very likely to evoke stress in most people. For example, research by investigators such as Seligman (1975), Janis and Mann (1979) and Schlenker and Leary (1982) has shown that stress is typically caused by:

- Threats to our self-concept or self-image and physical health.
- Situations involving conflict and ambiguity.
- Forced choices that have only unfavourable outcomes.
- Novel events that lead the individual to believe that the situational demands will outstrip their ability to cope.

Sometimes these factors interact. For example, conflict may arise when a patient has to make a forced choice between premature death and a disfiguring operation that threatens his or her body image. Additionally, the novel nature of the situation may cause the patient to question his or her ability to deal with the possible consequences of either course of action.

Dealing with stress

A number of factors mediate, or modify, the individual's response to threatening or challenging events. These include the levels of *social support* available to the individual and the individual's *personal coping mechanisms*. These two factors often interact, determining how well the individual copes with an event.

Social support

Social support mediates the stress response and the long-term damage that stress can cause. For example, social support has been shown to be important in protecting the individual from major illnesses such as heart disease, and in reducing morbidity and mortality post bereavement (Berkman 1995).

According to Cohen and Wills (1985), there are two basic ways in which social support may mediate the effects of stress. First, high levels of social support may prevent stress from occurring (the so-called *direct effect model*), because individuals with high levels of support are less likely to perceive challenging events as threatening. Second, social support may provide a cushion or buffer that protects the individuals from the most stressful aspects of challenging events (the so-called *buffering hypothesis*). So a well-supported individual that has been diagnosed as having, say, Parkinson's disease, is likely to experience less stress than an individual who lacks such support.

Social support may be offered in a variety of ways which can include:

• Emotional support.
• Self-esteem support
• Tangible or instrumental support.
• Network support.

Emotional and self-esteem support may be offered by the nurse during periods when the patient feels particularly low. Those experiencing depression, for example, often feel a sense of worthlessness that can be counteracted by someone spending time listening and talking to them. Similarly, the nurse can offer tangible support in the form of practical advice and information that may help to relieve stress by providing the patient with a means to deal with it. Whilst this type of support may normally be offered by friends and relatives, it is the *quality of support* rather than the size of the individual's network that is the critical factor in helping vulnerable individuals to meet their own needs (Schaefer *et al.* 1981).

Personal coping mechanisms

The extent to which individuals deal successfully or unsuccessfully with challenging situations is also determined by their *personal coping style* and their prior experience or *expectations* (Brewin 1988). Coping style may be loosely defined as habitual behaviour that is a function of the individual's personality traits or characteristics. For example, Type A individuals often view relatively neutral situations as competitive and threatening, and typically react to them with some hostility. Furthermore, the Type A's habitual behaviour may evoke feelings of competitiveness and guarded behaviour in his or her associates, which in turn serve to fuel the Type A's expectations, leading to continued hostile behaviour, and so on. (See Part Four for details of Type A-B behaviour.)

This cycle of events is not inevitable, and the nurse can help to alleviate the situation by being aware of, and checking, any feelings of hostility and competitiveness that are evoked by the patient's behaviour.

Personal control

Perhaps the single most important factor mediating reactions to potentially stressful events is the extent to which individuals believe that they have *control* over events. Research has shown, for example, that individuals high in *self-efficacy* have positive beliefs about their ability to adapt to new situations and to make things happen, have a greater sense of control or mastery over situations than those low in self-efficacy and tend to be less affected by stress (Bandura 1977; 1986). Similarly, individuals who possess the trait of *hardiness* have a sense of control over their lives, together with a sense of commitment and purpose that enables them to view change as a *positive challenge* rather than a threat (Kobasa 1979).

It has been suggested by *social learning* theorists that the belief in one's ability to master difficult situations is a trait-like characteristic that is formed during childhood (Bandura 1977; 1986). For example, individuals high in self-efficacy tend to have a high self-esteem and report memories of a happy childhood with caring and encouraging parents (Bee 1997). Whilst this finding fits well with the model of self-development outlined in Part One, it should be noted that children who display the trait of *resilience* (a characteristic very similar to hardiness) sometimes come from dysfunctional backgrounds where positive reinforcement and appropriate role models are not in evidence (Garmezy 1983; Hartrup 1983). This observation has led some researchers to argue that traits like self-efficacy, hardiness and resilience are, at least in part, a function of inherited personality characteristics (perhaps linked to the basic temperaments that we discussed in Part one).

Finally, it is worth noting that the illusory self-perceptions referred to earlier, such as denial, self-serving bias and downward social comparison, also serve to boost the individual's sense of personal control in addition to self-esteem.

Losing control: learned helplessness

According to *learned helplessness theory*, individuals lapse into a state of helplessness or depression as a result of situations where repeated efforts to exert control prove futile (Seligman 1975). However, there is more to it than this. Although it may seem rather paradoxical, it is often the patient's *perception* of control that is critical in determining a sense of helplessness, and not the gravity of the situation *per se*. For example, as noted earlier, cancer patients and their relatives sometimes possess an illusion of control that helps ward off feelings of helplessness even when the situation is dire (Taylor 1983). Conversely, it is possible for individuals to have a great deal of potential control over events, whilst believing that they have (and are exerting) almost none.

In the context of clinical practice, a loss of control may be experienced when important information about outcomes is withheld from the patient, because the threat of the unknown is often greater than the threat posed by reality (Hyland and Donaldson 1989). However, you also need to be aware that patients sometimes achieve a sense of control by ignoring or diluting reality, and in such cases it may be preferable to *withhold* information or to be especially sensitive and tentative about what is communicated.

Although it can sometimes be difficult to decide when to withhold or provide information about negative outcomes, the patient's verbal and non-verbal cues usually provide the necessary clues. However, such decisions do need to be taken carefully and are always aided by a good knowledge of the patient and a good relationship.

Adjustment to acute health crises

According to *crisis theory* (Caplan 1964), individuals faced with major threats to the self typically react by attempting to employ *tried and tested coping mechanisms*. If these work, the threat is diminished and the individual returns to a state of equilibrium. If, however, the use of tried and tested coping mechanisms fails, the individual responds by

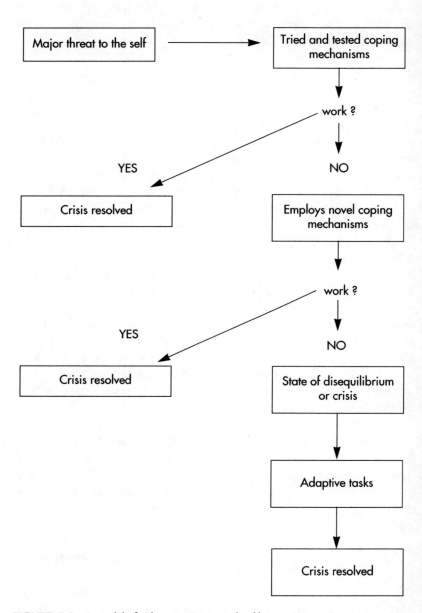

FIGURE 5.1 A model of adaptation to acute health crises

inventing new (and sometimes more desperate) ways of trying to deal with the event. As before, the threat is diminished if these *novel mechanisms* prove effective. If they fail, however, the individual enters a state of disequilibrium or *crisis*, typified by very high levels of anxiety, and resulting feelings of helplessness and despair (Benjamin 1978).

Caplan's model, which is shown schematically in Figure 5.1, is extremely useful and can be applied to explain acute stress reactions in *any* field of clinical practice. However, you should note that, unlike the learned helplessness model, Caplan's model is based on the premise that crises are naturally self-limiting, because the individual eventually *adapts* to the threat. Moos (1982) has taken this aspect of the model further, suggesting that patients experiencing an acute health crisis are typically faced with a number of *adaptive tasks* that they must accomplish if the crisis is to be resolved (see Figure 5.2). It seems reasonable to assume, therefore, that an individual will experience a sense of chronic helplessness and depression only if they are unable to complete these tasks successfully. It is relatively easy to envisage examples of the general and illness-related tasks suggested by Moos. For example, an inability to deal with pain might fuel the patient's anxiety and lead to the development of chronic and maladaptive pain behaviours (see Part Four). Similarly, the effects of trauma, surgery or a psychiatric diagnosis may render the individual unable to attain or preserve a satisfactory self-image, leading to a loss of self-esteem and feelings of depression.

Illness-related tasks

1 Dealing with pain, incapacitation and other symptoms
2 Dealing with the hospital environment and special treatment procedures
3 Developing and maintaining adequate relationships with health care staff

General tasks

4 Preserving a reasonable emotional balance
5 Preserving a satisfactory self-image
6 Preserving a relationship with family and friends
7 Preparing for an uncertain future.

FIGURE 5.2 Adaptive tasks associated with acute health crises, after Moos (1982)

Summary

The experience of stress is determined by:

- The nature or perceived severity of the challenging event.
- The individual's appraisal of what *it* will mean for them and how likely they are to deal with it successfully.
- Mediating factors such as social support, personal coping style and expectations.

A state of crisis may be evoked when:

- An individual perceives an event as threatening.
- Tried and tested coping responses and novel responses fail to diminish the perceived threat.
- The resulting response is one of very high anxiety and feelings of helplessness.

Chapter 6

Anxiety in clinical practice

Learning outcomes

By the end of this chapter you should be able to:

- Describe how classical conditioning may lead to the development of phobias and aversive reactions.
- Describe the causes and consequences of anxiety in hospitals.
- Outline the basic features of post-traumatic stress disorder.

The nature of anxiety

Anxiety is a common reaction that arises when individuals believe that their physical or psychological well-being is threatened, and in this respect anxiety is an integral part of the normal stress response. However, stress and anxiety are treated as unique constructs, because of the existence of specific anxiety disorders that are not regarded as part of the normal reaction to stress. These disorders include phobias and post traumatic stress disorder. A knowledge of these disorders and their aetiology is important because they are relatively common, and invasive clinical procedures may serve to trigger them.

Phobias

A phobia may be defined as an *irrational fear* that is out of proportion to the actual threat posed to the individual. It is typically characterised by *avoidance* of the eliciting stimulus and is often accompanied by feelings of *panic* (Mowrer 1947). For example, individuals who are claustrophobic may actively avoid lifts and other enclosed spaces that lead them to feel anxious and panicky.

Many phobias, such as arachnophobia (a fear of spiders), result in high levels of anxiety only when the eliciting stimulus is in close proximity, and since the offending stimulus can often be easily avoided, they tend not to be overly disruptive. However, certain phobias may be triggered by stimuli or events that are difficult to avoid without causing marked inhibition of normal social activities. For example, individuals who suffer from *agoraphobia* (from the Greek word meaning fear of market places) typically become very anxious and panicky when they find themselves in public settings, such as supermarkets and buses. This fear eventually leads afflicted individuals to cocoon themselves in a place of safety, which often results in them being unable to leave their homes without experiencing intense anxiety. It is this disruptive element combined with the accompanying anxiety that often prompts individuals to seek professional help (Marks 1987).

Specific phobias

Specific phobias form the single most common class of phobia, and, as the name suggests, the phobic response is elicited by specific stimuli, such as spiders, wasps, heights, the sight of blood, etc. This class of phobia is quite common. For example, Agras (1969) found that approximately seventy-seven in every 1,000 individuals reported a phobia related to a specific event or object. However, only two to three individuals in every 1,000 reported that the phobia was severe and disabling.

Whilst there are numerous theories that seek to explain how phobias develop, the most widely accepted is based upon *learning or behavioural theory*. According to this school of thought, a phobia develops when a previously neutral stimulus is paired closely in time with an event that results in some considerable trauma involving anxiety, pain, or nausea (Rosenhan and Seligman 1995).

In order to understand this, we might imagine a scenario where a young toddler experiences a sharp, burning pain immediately after seeing a wasp on his arm. According to learning theory, this event would result in the toddler learning to associate the wasp with pain, because the two events (the sight of the insect and the feeling of pain) were paired closely in time. Although we might well imagine that such events would always result in the development of a phobia if the event was sufficiently traumatic, this is not always the case. Indeed, exactly why one individual may develop only mild anxiety following a traumatic or aversive event, whilst another may develop a phobia, is something of a puzzle. However, studies have shown that children are at a higher risk of developing specific types of phobia if one of their parents is also a sufferer (Cromer 1996). It has been argued that this suggests a genetic link, but, as we will see later, there are alternative explanations.

An occasional, but important, feature of phobia acquisition involves the *generalisation* of the fear to other similar stimuli (Marks 1987). For example, a toddler's fear of wasps may generalise to a fear of all insects that look or sound something like wasps. This does not occur in all cases, but where it does, it increases the potential for inhibition of normal social activities.

Experimental proof of this model of phobia acquisition was offered by Watson and Rayner (1928). They induced a phobia in an 11-month-old boy, 'little Albert', by repeatedly pairing the presentation of a white rat (to which the child initially showed only curiosity) with a loud and disturbing noise. After a number of pairings, the mere sight of the rat evoked feelings of fear in the child, and this response eventually generalised to other classes of rodent (and allegedly to fur coats and toys). Although highly unethical, the case study does offer support for the position that phobic reactions can be induced by pairing a previously neutral stimulus with a traumatic or aversive event.

Classical conditioning and phobia acquisition

Classical conditioning theory is based on the premise that learning occurs when a neutral stimulus is paired with a biologically significant event that may be either pleasant or aversive. In order to understand what this actually means, and how it relates to phobia acquisition, we will briefly examine some of the theory's basic tenets.

Basic classical conditioning theory

Whilst it is a normal reflexive action for hungry dogs to salivate when they smell food, Pavlov (1927) discovered that dogs in his laboratory would salivate in *anticipation* of being fed, following the presentation of certain non-biological cues in the dogs' environment. He experimented further and developed a theory to account for this phenomenon, which may be explained using *classical conditioning* shorthand (see Figure 6.1). During Stage 1, the dogs respond to the smell of meat by salivating. The meat is termed the unconditioned stimulus (UCS), meaning that it is a naturally occurring stimulus, and the response, salivation, is termed the unconditioned response (UCR), because it also occurs naturally. During Stage 2, a conditioned stimulus (CS), such as a bell, repeatedly precedes the UCS, and during this *acquisition phase* the animals learn to *associate* the two events with each other. During Stage 3, learning is complete, and presentation of the CS alone results in a conditioned or learned response (CR).

Originally, learning theorists argued that learning took place during the acquisition phase simply because the CS and UCS were repeatedly paired closely in time. This was revised, however, following evidence that suggested that learning occurs because the presence of the CS allows the animal to *predict* the event that is about to occur (Rescorla 1967). That is, the animal learns that the occurrence of the significant event is *contingent* upon the presence of the conditioned stimulus. This

Stage 1

UCS   (meat) . . . .   UCR
(salivation)

Stage 2

CS (bell) UCS . . . . . acquisition phase . . . .   X trials

Stage 3

CS   . . . .   CR
(salivation)

FIGURE 6.1 Learning by classical conditioning

has led to the hypothesis that the CS acts as a signal that an important event (pleasant or unpleasant) is about to occur. More specifically, the CS may act as either a *danger signal* or a *safety signal*, depending upon the circumstances (Seligman 1975).

The apparent importance of danger signals was illustrated in an experiment conducted by Weiss (1972). In his experiment, rats in the 'warning condition' were given electric shocks preceded by a ten second warning tone. Rats in the 'no warning condition' were given identical and simultaneous shocks, but were given no prior warning of when the shock would occur. Weiss found that the rats in the no warning condition quickly developed extensive ulceration, whilst rats in the warning condition were relatively unharmed. This finding suggested to Weiss that the absence of a danger signal made it impossible for the rats in the no warning condition to know when their environment was safe, and the resultant state of chronic high arousal led to severe physiological damage.

Atkinson *et al.* (1993) state that the presence of danger signals is important in clinical settings too. For example, they argue that if a doctor administering an injection tells a young child that it will hurt a little, the syringe becomes a danger signal that signals anxiety, and this continues until the agent is administered and the needle is put away. Let us ask, though, what would happen if the doctor tells the child that the injection will not hurt and it subsequently does? Although we cannot be sure, it seems likely that the *doctor* would become the danger signal, which would result in anxiety whenever the child visited the doctor.

In extreme cases, it is possible that such an event could lead to the development of a phobia, and this position is broadly supported by anecdotal research. For example, Tuma and Masser (1985) found that phobia acquisition was made more likely by unpredictable events, and Scott and Glum (1984) found that phobia development in patients was made less likely when patients were provided with prior information about treatment procedures.

It is worth noting that whilst objects such as syringes may act as danger signals, the presence of certain objects or people can act as reassuring safety signals. For example, children generally associate their parents with comfort and reassurance, and their presence during aversive clinical procedures generally helps to convey a feeling of safety to the child.

Phobia extinction

According to classical conditioning theory, when a CS no longer heralds a significant pleasant or aversive event, the learning based upon the original CS–UCS contingency is extinguished over time. Say, for example, the rats in Weiss's warning condition had been subsequently exposed to the warning tone with no resulting shock, they would have eventually learned to ignore the tone, because it offered no useful information. Similarly, if an individual has developed a fear of going to the dentist that has resulted from repeated pairings of injections of local anaesthetic (CS) with the dentist (UCS), the learned fear response would gradually extinguish over time if the dentist developed a new pain-killing technique that did not involve administering injections. This would occur because the presence of the CS no longer signalled or predicted pain.

Imagine, however, that an individual had developed a phobia of dentists so intense that he never kept any appointments. Would we expect the phobia to extinguish over time? The answer to this is no. The phobia would remain in place because the original CS–UCS contingency link would remain in his memory. Put another way, the avoidance helps to maintain the phobia, as the expectation that visits to the dentist result in painful injections is never challenged.

Finally, it is important to note that individuals typically know that their phobias are irrational, but are unable to correct them by logical thinking or persuasion. This suggests that learning by association takes place in some phylogentically primitive part of the brain. In fact, successful treatments for phobias typically involve challenging the phobia by direct experience rather than reason, by employing thera- peutic techniques such as *flooding* and *systematic desensitisation*. If you are interested in learning more about these treatments, I would encourage you to refer to the texts by Davidson and Neale (1994) and Rosenhan and Seligman (1995) cited in the References (p. 209).

Classical conditioning and adverse reactions in clinical practice

Whilst traumatic events do not necessarily lead to phobia acquisition, they can lead to classically conditioned responses that can be equally aversive and undesirable. (It should be noted that classically conditioned reactions, such as taste aversion or anticipatory nausea are not classified as phobic reactions, because they may occur in the absence of the high levels of anxiety that are associated with phobias.) Indeed, given that many clinical procedures are invasive and potentially traumatic, it is possible that individual patients might come to associate previously neutral stimuli in the clinical environment with traumatic procedures involving pain, nausea, etc. In fact, there is some evidence that this can occur in clinical practice. For example, Melamed and Siegel (1985) found that children undergoing treatment for cancer may develop aversive responses, such as vomiting, on mere exposure to hospital settings. This might plausibly occur as follows: first the chemotherapy agent (UCS) and nausea (UCR) become associated with the smell of the hospital (CS), and over time this association results in conditioned nausea (CR) on mere exposure to the hospital. There is some evidence to support this hypothesis. For example, Coons *et al.* (1990) state that nausea can come to be associated with the venipuncture procedure used to administer chemotherapy agents, so that *anticipatory nausea* occurs at the mere sight of the needle or cannula. It appears that children are particularly likely to develop aversive reactions and that these often involve nausea as the unconditioned response. Douglas and Byron (1996), for example, report that severe eating difficulties in children are often associated with a prior history of frequent vomiting, gagging or tube feeding, which leads to a fear and avoidance of solid foods.

Although classical conditioning reactions typically occur only after repeated CS-UCS pairings, there is evidence that conditioned reactions may occur following a single traumatic or biologically salient pairing. For example, Davidson and Foa (1993) found that classically conditioned taste aversion in dogs can occur after a one-off ingestion of inedible food that has resulted in vomiting. Presumably, the significance of this event is registered immediately, because it would be potentially hazardous to ingest the same type of food for a second time. As this suggests that biologically significant or traumatic events can result in classical conditioning on the basis of a single episode, it is feasible that patients may develop adverse reactions rapidly when the response involves biologically salient stimuli, such as pain or nausea.

Whilst the limited evidence available suggests that making patients aware of the likelihood of adverse outcomes may offer some protection, the very nature of traumatic events means that they cannot always be anticipated. It is, therefore, important that the nurse should be aware of the potential for aversive reactions in vulnerable patients, of whom the most susceptible are probably young children.

Alternative models

The classical conditioning model is not without its critics, because only a small proportion of adverse reactions or phobias can be traced to the occurrence of traumatic events (Lazarus 1971). Furthermore, as mentioned earlier, classical conditioning theory cannot satisfactorily explain why a traumatic event may lead to the development of a phobia in one individual and only mild anxiety in another.

These and other problems have led to alternative explanations being sought for the development of phobias and aversive reactions. It has been shown, for example, that direct experience of an aversive event is not necessary for the development of a phobia. Instead, learning may occur by simple observation, which is termed *vicarious reinforcement* (Bandura 1986). For example, a child may develop a fear of spiders simply by observing his mother's own terrified response to spiders, and Melamed and Siegel (1985) argue that phobic reactions in children undergoing treatment for cancer may be acquired through observation of their parents' anxious responses. If this model of acquisition is correct, it is possible that phobic reactions could develop in children as young as 10 months of age, as it has been shown that at around this stage children reliably begin to show signs of distress when their mother's facial expression reflects anxiety (Dickstein and Parke 1988).

Research into learning theory and phobia acquisition is complex and is riddled with theoretical issues that have not yet been satisfactorily resolved. However, the most important points to glean from the discussion so far are that traumatic events may cause adverse reactions, of which the patient has little or no control, and that the likelihood of such reactions occurring may be reduced by preparing the patient, wherever possible, for aversive or traumatic clinical procedures or events.

Post traumatic stress disorder

Post traumatic stress disorder (or PTSD) is a severe and protracted stress reaction that is triggered by catastrophic or traumatic events. It can have a lasting effect on individuals, leaving them with a deep-seated fear and a feeling that another catastrophe is waiting just around the corner.

PTSD has been described as a broad collection of symptoms that together form a complex syndrome (see Figure 6.2). For example, PTSD shares a number of the features inherent in phobias, such as the feelings of panic and anxiety that occur when an individual is exposed to triggering cues (Marks 1987). Yet it is also characterised by persistently high levels of arousal, and by emotions, such as anger, depression and self-blame, that are atypical of phobic reactions (Joseph *et al.* 1997). Because PTSD is such a complex disorder, a number of theoretical frameworks have been applied to try and explain how it is caused and how the reaction is maintained. For example, it has been suggested that PTSD may be caused by a sudden and overwhelming loss of control evoking learned helplessness, and classical conditioning has been used to explain why internal and external stimuli can trigger symptoms long after the event has occurred. Perhaps the most intriguing explanation, however, stems from ideas proposed by Horowitz (1975) and Joseph *et al.* (1997).

According to the latter authors, people live in a 'bubble of perceived invulnerability' (Joseph *et al.* 1997, p. 1), believing that they are immune to events such as floods, criminal assault, fires, etc. (you may recognise the links here with illusory self-perceptions). In the case of PTSD, this bubble is violently punctured by an event that is beyond the limits of normal human experience. Horowitz (1975) argues that this results in a profound sense of disequilibrium, as the individual's schematic view of the world is shattered. In turn, this leads to an intense sense of vulnerability and a flooding of attention and memory with intrusive thoughts, images and emotions. If the event is sufficiently traumatic, the individual may be unable to process these emotions, and is thus forced persistently to 'relive' the incident, because the event cannot be removed from the forefront of conscious awareness.

Using this framework, we may ascertain that *any* traumatic event has the potential to evoke PTSD, if it is severe enough to shatter the individual's sense of invulnerability. This is an important point, because we tend to think of PTSD as being linked only to large-scale disasters that occur infrequently. However, Joseph *et al.* (1997) point out that relatively common, and sometimes highly personal, events can trigger PTSD, such as road traffic accidents, childhood sexual abuse and adult rape. In addition, there is evidence of its occurrence in medical settings. For example, Goldbeck-Wood (1996) reports that PTSD in mothers may result from traumatic childbirth, and Alter *et al.* (1996) found evidence of PTSD in a sample of cancer patients at up to three years from the time of the original diagnosis. Similarly, Pelcovitz *et al.* (1996) found that mothers of children with cancer were at a significantly increased risk of PTSD compared to women in a control group, and Butler *et al.* (1996) found evidence of PTSD in children receiving treatment for cancer.

- Person is exposed to a traumatic event involving horror, fear and helplessness.

- Event is constantly recurring by way of images, thoughts, perceptions, nightmares, repetitive play in children, flashbacks and intense distress on exposure to triggering cues.

- Evidence of avoidance of stimuli and places associated with the event.

- Emotional blunting and/or intense emotions, such as anger, anxiety, guilt and shame.

- Persistent symptoms of arousal, such as insomnia, irritability, impaired concentration and exaggerated startle response.

FIGURE 6.2 Core features of PTSD, adapted from DSM IV (1994)

As with most stress-related reactions, PTSD is mediated by social support and by personal coping mechanisms, such as the trait of hardiness. Furthermore, Rosenhan and Seligman (1995) state that predisposing genetic factors, the individual's prior state of mental health and prior experiences, can all render the individual more, or less, vulnerable to the effects of highly stressful events.

Finally, you should note that although traumatic events such as emergency surgery are, by their very nature, difficult to predict and avoid, many medical interventions are planned in advance. So, given that one of the precipitating factors in PTSD is uncontrollability, it makes sense to prepare patients for potentially aversive outcomes wherever possible.

Anxiety and stress in hospitals

Although we do not have an accurate estimate of how many hospitalised patients come to be severely traumatised, I would hazard a guess that the numbers are fairly low. This is not to underestimate the aversive nature of many types of illness and treatments, or to suggest that we should not be concerned about the potential for PTSD , but it is an acknowledgement that, in many cases, trauma is neither totally overwhelming nor unexpected. This said, it is important to remember that anxiety is a common response to hospitalisation, and that even admission for routine investigations can evoke relatively high levels of anxiety in patients (Johnston and Wallace 1990). Given this, it is obviously important to recognise signs of stress in patients and to be aware of the types of event that individuals are likely to find anxiety-provoking. According to Pitts (1991), the following categories of event are particularly likely to elicit anxiety and stress:

- Being in a novel situation that involves a reversal or loss of normal social roles.
- Loss of control and depersonalisation.
- The prospect of surgery, including losing control, not regaining consciousness, being cut and feeling pain during the procedure and post-operatively.
- Separation from family and friends.
- Lack of normal 'distracting' activities.
- Inadequate levels of communication.

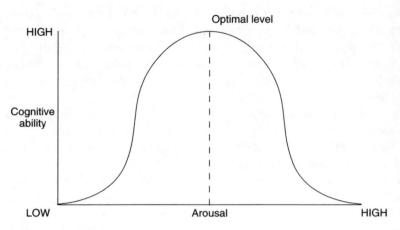

FIGURE 6.3 The Yerkes-Dodson Law

Anxiety can have a marked effect on our ability to process, store and recall information. In small doses, anxiety actually *improves* the individual's cognitive performance, but at high levels overall performance is significantly impaired. This apparent paradox was explained by Yerkes and Dodson (1908), who formulated a law showing that the relationship between cognitive ability and levels of autonomic arousal follows a typical inverted U shape (see Figure 6.3).

It is easy to conceptualise this law in action. Imagine having to sit an important assessment minutes after you have just woken up, with no caffeine to boost your system, or try and recall an event (like an important interview or date) where your actions have been clumsy and uncoordinated despite your best efforts. Now imagine yourself as, say, an elderly patient being admitted for diagnostic tests on a busy ward with a hassled nurse giving you rushed instructions. Put this way, the end result is rather obvious. Unfortunately, when confusion and 'loss of memory' are seen in elderly patients, it is all too often attributed to old age. In fact, as we will learn shortly, research does not support the stereotype that elderly people are all cognitively challenged (Birren and Schaie 1990), though there is evidence that their cognitive ability is more likely to be affected by anxiety than that of, say, middle-aged adults (Woods and Britton 1985).

Whatever the differences caused by age, it is important to remember that hospitals are generally perceived as unfamiliar and stressful environments, which can evoke anxiety, and associated confusion, in all age groups.

Summary

Whilst transient anxiety is a normal response to novel or challenging situations, traumatic events can trigger a range of adverse reactions, which include phobias, anticipatory nausea and post traumatic stress disorder.

It is difficult to gauge the extent or frequency of occurrence of such events in clinical practice, because relatively little research has been carried out. However, the limited evidence available suggests that such reactions may be mediated by providing the patient with prior information about potentially aversive outcomes, such as pain and nausea. A failure to do so may place the patient in an unpredictable situation that lacks obvious danger or safety signals. The stress that this causes is likely to have a deleterious effect on the patient's physical and psychological health which, animal experiments suggest, could be serious in extreme circumstances.

Chapter 7

Anger and aggression in clinical practice

Learning outcomes

By the end of this chapter you should be able to:

- Describe the nature of anger and aggression.
- Describe the basic causes of emotional aggression.
- Outline how aggression may be avoided in clinical practice.

Anger and aggression in clinical practice

Aggression towards nurses and other health professionals is relatively commonplace, with most incidents occurring in the areas of psychiatry, learning disabilities, accident and emergency and elderly care (Wykes 1994). Although aggression is stereotypically associated with young males and excessive alcohol, the likelihood of aggression is increased in *all* population groups as a consequence of factors associated with illness. In order to understand the reasons for this, we will examine the basic causes of anger and aggression, before exploring what can be done to minimise them.

The nature of anger and aggression

Berkowitz (1993) states that *anger* is an unpleasant feeling that results from internal, physiological states, whilst aggression is a behavioural act that has two basic forms: *hostile aggression*, which is equated with a deliberate and premeditated attempt to hurt someone physically or psychologically, and *emotional aggression*, which is associated with an impulsive act that results from high and aversive levels of physiological arousal. According to Berkowitz, most acts of aggression fall into the latter category, occurring spontaneously when the normal threshold for aggression is lowered as a result of considerable pressure and frustration. Indeed, according to the Frustration–Aggression hypothesis (Dollard *et al.* 1939), aggression is often linked to *frustration* caused by the *blocking of personal goals* and it represents a desire to regain a sense of control (May 1972). Given this context, it is relatively easy to understand how illness and hospitalisation can lead to emotional aggression, compounded by factors such as pain, long waiting periods, separation from loved ones, noise, loss of privacy and reversal of normal social roles (Letemendia 1985; Wright 1985).

Berkowitz argues that frustration initially leads to attempts to avoid the stressor and to the development of alternative goals.

However, when repeated attempts at overcoming blocks eventually prove futile, frustration builds to such a level that emotional aggression is almost inevitable. Weiner (1986) states this is most likely to happen when the causal event is viewed as *intentional*, *avoidable* and *malevolent*. Viewed from this attributional perspective, it is easy to understand why a football player, tackled from behind every time he approaches the goal, eventually erupts into a display of overt aggression, and why, by the same token, a patient waiting for a long time in casualty is less likely to be aggressive towards staff if she perceives that they are struggling to deal with the aftermath of a major incident. However, Weiner's attributional framework is less likely to be applicable when the patient's thought processes are clouded by factors such as intense pain, alcohol, medication or psychotic illness.

It is important to note that, according to Miller (1941) and Davitz (1952), the ultimate aim of aggression is not always to hurt the victim. For example, aggression may have the goal of

1   restoring a negative self-concept and changing one's social status (as when a gang member inflicts injury on an innocent victim to gain 'prestige');
2   attaining a sense of power and control (as when a senior member of staff suffering from low self-esteem 'puts down' a junior colleague in order to get a temporary ego boost); and
3   removing a stressor that is blocking one's goals (as may occur when a dementing patient lashes out because he is embarrassed at or frightened of being undressed by 'strangers').

- High levels of internal, physiological arousal associated with anxiety and stress
- Frustration due to blocked goals, particularly if the event is perceived as intentional, avoidable and malevolent
- A sense of powerlessness and loss of control
- Pain, alcohol, medication and psychotic illnesses that lower the normal aggression threshold
- Low self-esteem

FIGURE 7.1 Factors that make emotional aggression more likely

In short, illness and hospitalisation often provide the conditions that foster emotional aggression. Some of the factors that make it more likely are listed in Figure 7.1.

Avoiding or preventing emotional aggression

In view of the fact that most acts of aggression result from emotional stress, we need to explore how we can reduce the stressors associated with hospitalisation and illness. Wright (1985) argues that illness reminds us of our vulnerability and personal inadequacies, and the sense of powerlessness that this may evoke can lead to primitive, instinctual urges to escape or regain control through aggression. Consequently, aggression can sometimes be avoided by the implementation of nursing practices that seek to reduce feelings of helplessness. This may be achieved at a basic level by providing the patient with information or activities that foster a sense of control. This basic rule applies to everyone. If, for example, you have ever been left waiting for a bus or train to arrive with no available information, you will know that it is the lack of information, rather than the delay *per se*, that creates the sense of powerlessness and frustration.

Of course, it is not always possible to prevent these feelings when illness strikes, so there are good arguments for permitting some expression of anger, perhaps through just being an available 'listening vent'. Unfortunately, this basic need is sometimes overlooked in clinical practice. Skynner and Cleese (1983) suggest that the need to avoid anger may stem from childhood experiences where many families view it (and sometimes other powerful emotions too) as negative and un-desirable. Alternative outlets for anger and aggression can sometimes be achieved by what Freud (1901) termed *sublimation* or the channelling of socially unacceptable behaviour into appropriate activities. For example, hospitalised patients may benefit from physical exercise and other forms of activity, where they are fit enough to do so.

In general terms, we may state that giving patients permission to vent their frustration is desirable, provided that it does not adversely affect others. Furthermore, Letemendia (1985) argues that it is important that the nurse does not respond to aggression with corresponding anger. This may be achieved by stepping back and viewing the patient's position objectively rather than subjectively, and by focusing on the conditions that underpin the patient's behaviour rather than the behaviour itself. Patients whose cognitions are clouded by pain, medication or psychotic illness need a special approach that seeks to avoid compounding internal levels of arousal, by providing a calm milieu, free from excessive noise and other stimuli that might overload the individual. In short, there is a great deal the nurse can do to alleviate aggression in clinical practice.

Summary

Anger may be broadly defined as an unpleasant state of physiological arousal, and aggression as a behavioural act that results in some sort of emotional release. Unlike hostile aggression, emotional aggression is typically impulsive, and any injury inflicted on a third party is often secondary to primary goals, such as a need to regain a sense of control, a need to remove a stressor or a need to boost a low self-esteem. Aggression is also made more likely if events blocking personal goals are perceived as being intentional, avoidable and malevolent. Furthermore, factors such as pain, alcohol and medication may reduce the normal threshold that inhibits aggressive acts.

It is possible to reduce or avoid aggression in clinical practice by utilising strategies that enhance self-esteem and provide the individual with a sense of control. In addition, it is important to provide appropriate outlets for anger wherever possible. Patients who are confused or psychotic generally benefit from being nursed in a quiet, calm environment that avoids exacerbating the high levels of internal arousal that often accompany these states.

Chapter 8

Depression in clinical practice

Learning outcomes

By the end of this chapter you should be able to:

- Describe the basic causes and consequences of depression.
- Recognise the basic features of depression.
- Indicate how basic aspects of nursing care can benefit the individual with depression.

Causes and consequences of depression

There can be few adults that have not heard of depression and even fewer that have not experienced times when they have felt low in mood. Yet, despite its commonalty, depression is a phenomenon that defies simple definition. This is largely because it spans a continuum that ranges from a normal and transient response to events involving personal disappointment and loss, through to an abnormal mood disorder that may lack an obvious cause and which may require prolonged psychological or medical intervention (Davidson and Neale 1994). Similarly, the symptoms of depression can vary markedly, and range from a mild and transient state of 'the blues' to a persistent and disabling condition that pervades all aspects of the individual's emotional, cognitive and behavioural functioning. This latter form is normally labelled *clinical depression*, and it is estimated that approximately twelve in every 100 people will experience at least one episode of depression during their life time that is serious enough to warrant this label and some form of professional help (Cromer 1996).

Depression may be *reactive*, or psychological, in origin, arising in response to some life event or loss, or it may be *endogenous*, or internal, in origin, arising as a by-product of some underlying metabolic disturbance or disease process. This distinction is sometimes blurred in clinical practice. For example, according to the biological, or medical, model, the depression often present in the early stages of Alzheimer's disease is a consequence of altered brain chemistry caused by the disease process itself, whilst according to the psychological model, the depression is a function of the individual's awareness of his or her inability to function normally and a sense that something is dreadfully wrong (Lancaster 1984).

Of course, it is feasible that depression may result as an interaction of *both* psychological and physiological processes, and it is, therefore, wise to bear this in mind when dealing with any depressed patient who is known to have some underlying organic condition.

Although depression is undoubtedly most prevalent in psychiatric populations, there has been a tendency to underestimate its occurrence in general medical settings. The Royal College of Physicians and Psychiatrists (1995), for example, has estimated that depression occurs in approximately 12–16 per cent of medical patients, with a much higher rate (25–35 per cent) in severe acute and disabling chronic illnesses involving, for example, cancer, heart disease, rheumatoid arthritis and cerebral haemorrhage or strokes. These worrying figures prompted the college to recommend that urgent action be taken to ensure that doctors and nurses are given the skills to detect and treat depression more effectively.

Recognising and dealing with depression

Detecting depression in clinical practice can be a tricky business, not least because it is sometimes difficult to know when to regard an episode of depression as normal and expected and when to treat it as abnormal and severe. Whilst this problem does not apply so much in the field of mental health, where depression is often severe and easily detected, it does apply to general medical and community settings, where episodes of depression are often milder and where there is a prior *expectation* that many patients receiving secondary or tertiary treatments for illness will be upset and low for periods of time. In both cases, the question is not so much *whether* the patient needs some form of support, as *what* needs to be offered and by whom.

In general terms, milder episodes of depression often result in response to actual or anticipated loss. Furthermore, the processes triggered are often self-limiting and require little more than time for adjustment and the presence of an available, sympathetic listener to speed things towards a natural conclusion. There are exceptions to this rule, however, and they generally apply to events where individuals have extreme difficulty adjusting to change or loss. Recently bereaved individuals, for example, can become very depressed, and there is no consensus of opinion as to whether such episodes warrant formal interventions, such as counselling or anti-depressant medication, or whether the event should be allowed to run its own natural course. Indeed, as we will learn shortly, it is possible to imagine many different types of scenario where patients experience, or anticipate, some sort of loss that results in depression as part and parcel of the adjustment process.

In borderline cases, specific diagnostic criteria can help the psychiatrist or psychologist to decide whether or not an individual's depression is sufficiently severe as to warrant expert help. Figure 8.1 shows one such set of criteria adapted from DSM IV (1994). As a rule, a diagnosis of depression is made only if several core symptoms are present for a period of fourteen days or longer, though most clinicians supplement formal diagnostic criteria with their knowledge of the patient and his or her circumstances.

As a nurse, it is unlikely that you will be asked formally to diagnose depression, but as you have a great deal of contact with patients, you are able to play an invaluable role in detecting the basic signs and symptoms in vulnerable individuals, with a view to offering immediate support or to referring the patient on to an appropriate agency. To do this effectively, you need good observation skills, a good relationship with your patient or client, and a knowledge of the core symptoms of depression. In instances where you are unsure whether a patient needs expert help, it may help to table the following questions and discuss your conclusions with your team or a knowledgeable colleague:

- What specific symptoms have I observed (e.g. low mood, apathy, insomnia, etc.)?
- Are the symptoms a response to an identifiable event, involving loss or change?
- Do the patient's symptoms appear abnormally severe in consideration of the event?
- How many days have the symptoms been present?

- Sad depressed mood
- Negative self-concept and low self-esteem
- Poor levels of concentration and difficulty thinking
- Feelings of guilt, worthlessness and anger
- Loss of interest in normal activities
- Loss of sleep, disturbed sleep or excessive sleep
- Poor appetite/weight loss or weight gain (or failure to make expected weight gains in children)
- Lethargy or agitation
- Recurrent thoughts about death and suicide

FIGURE 8.1 The core features of depression, adapted from DSM IV (1994)

Theories of depression

Learned helplessness theory

According to *learned helplessness theory*, individuals exposed to uncontrollable events initially react against the stressor by expressing anger, but on realising that their efforts are futile, eventually lapse into a state of apathy that is marked by a loss of motivation, feelings of helplessness and an overall decline in cognitive functioning (Seligman 1975). These features closely mimic the core characteristics of clinical depression.

The original learned helplessness theory provided a powerful, yet simple, explanation of depression, and it was easy to envisage why events associated with depression, such as illness and bereavement, could evoke learned helplessness. However, the theory was subsequently modified to deal with a number of theoretical anomalies, which included the realisation that the individual's perception of control was often more important than the actual levels of control available in any given situation (as you may recall from our discussions of cancer patients and coping in Part One). Furthermore, subsequent research showed that, as a rule, individuals develop depression only if they attribute some untoward event to *internal, global* and *stable factors* (Abramson *et al.* 1978). This is not as complicated as it might sound. Imagine, for example, a situation where a young student nurse fails an important exam. In seeking to understand the event, she may first attribute the failure to internal factors and chastise herself for a lack of ability or a weak will. Second, she may attribute failure to global factors, inferring that everything she does is lacking. Third, she may attribute failure to stable factors, viewing the failure as one of a series of past and future failures. In short, if the student blames herself for the failure, views it as a symptom of a general lack of ability and perceives it as a consistent problem that is likely to be encountered every time she has to pass an assessment, she is at a high risk of experiencing depression.

Interestingly, there is some evidence that females are more likely to attribute failure to internal factors than males, whilst males are more likely than their female counterparts to make an external attribution and blame others or other things (Deaux 1984). It has been suggested that these differences are due to the passive role that young females are expected to adopt in a male-dominated world, and this may go some way to explaining why women are at a higher risk of developing depression than males. In younger populations, the validity of this stereotype is questionable (certainly, many of the female students I come across are very forceful in their assertions that this is definitely *not* the role adopted by 1990s woman!). However, the stereotype may be valid for those most at risk of developing depression, namely those who are aged 50 plus (Davidson and Neale 1994).

A final revision to learned helplessness theory is based on evidence that some individuals consistently view themselves, and life, in a negative way. This trait-like, pessimistic outlook is associated with a sense of hopelessness and an increased risk of depression (Metalsky *et al.* 1987) that, as we will see next, has much in common with the belief that depression is caused by a negative cognitive set, or 'faulty thinking'.

The faulty thinking view of depression

Whereas 'normal' individuals seek to boost their self-esteem via positive illusory self-perceptions, such as the self-serving bias (see Part One), Beck (1976; 1987) has argued that depressed individuals tend to:

- Magnify their failures and minimise their successes.
- Over-generalise the effects of failure.
- Focus selectively on certain (negative) events.

In fact, the most important aspect of Beck's theory is its premise that an individual's thinking can *cause* depression. This view is radically different from the stance that the individual is a passive being that becomes depressed as a consequence of uncontrollable stressors or biological events. Furthermore, Beck's thinking led to the creation of *cognitive therapies* for depression, wherein individuals are alerted to cognitive distortions in their patterns of thinking and are challenged to correct them.

A model of depression

Figure 8.2 shows a simplified model of depression that may help you to integrate the presented concepts and theories into a straightforward framework. According to the model, there are four basic causes of depression: life events, severance of attachments, faulty thinking and biological events.

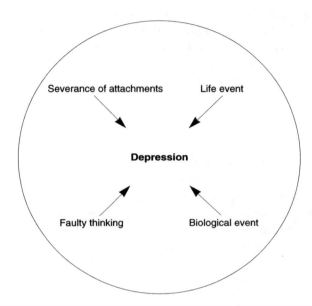

FIGURE 8.2 A model of the causes of depression

Life events

Major life events, such as bereavement, illness or redundancy, can cause depression when the individual no longer possesses a *sense of control* or mastery over events, and when there is an *absence of social support* and/or a *loss of social status* (Brown and Harris 1978). Such events can cause the individual to feel vulnerable and to react with initial anxiety or anger (as in the flight-fright response), before deploying coping mechanisms such as denial or projection (see Part One) in an effort to reduce the severity of the threat. If such attempts at coping fail, the individual may come to experience a sense of helplessness or hopelessness that eventually leads to a state of depression (Caplan 1964; Seligman 1975).

Severance of attachments

According to Bowlby (1980), the death of someone or something close to us leads to the *severance of a cherished emotional bond* or attachment that evokes a profound sense of loss. This can also be understood with reference to Cooley's (1902) proposal that people close to us gradually become integrated into our self-concept over time, so that their loss is represented internally as the loss of an important part of the self, which results in a strong sense of emptiness, hopelessness and depression.

Faulty thinking

Some individuals have a negative self-image and a pessimistic outlook which leads them to distort reality in line with their expectations. The resultant *faulty thinking* perpetuates their negative self-image and renders them prone to major depressive episodes (Beck 1976).

Research has offered some support for Beck's hypothesis. For example, depressed people typically attribute successes to external factors and failures to internal factors (Rosenhan and Seligman 1995). As noted earlier, this is a reverse of the self-serving bias, wherein individuals typically attribute success to internal factors and failures to external factors. We can sum this up by stating that depression appears to be associated with negative biases in information-processing, whilst mental health appears to be associated with positive biases in information-processing.

Biological events

It is important to note that whilst depression may result from faulty, or negative, thinking, as Beck suggests, it is quite feasible that adverse life events could lead to depression, and any resultant negative thinking might be construed as entirely realistic and appropriate. Furthermore, it is conceivable that faulty thinking may result from internal biological factors, such as cancer, old age, metabolic disturbance and intra-cranial events, which may alter the subtle balance of *neurotransmitters* such as *serotonin* in the brain, thus precipitating depression (Bunney *et al.* 1970).

Focus on clinical practice: the myth of ageing and inevitable decline

Regardless of age, the ability to cope successfully with life's trials and tribulations is dependent upon our resourcefulness, our beliefs about our ability to deal with whatever life throws at us, and our physical status, which sets limits on what we can or cannot hope to achieve. In short, the effective coper is likely to be intelligent and resourceful, high in self-esteem and physically fit. It is, therefore, unfortunate that in our society elderly people are often portrayed as lacking in these characteristics and are, instead, stereotypically labelled as inflexible, lacking in intelligence and physically frail. Yet research suggests that this damning picture is something of a myth perpetrated by misconceptions about the general effects of ageing on intelligence, personality and physical well-being.

In the following section we will focus on these issues and show that the elderly are generally as well placed to cope with adverse events as any other group in society (barring the effects of socio-economic factors that are beyond the scope of this handbook).

Cognitive ability and age

During the 1970s, researchers using standardised intelligence or IQ tests found evidence that appeared to show that cognitive ability declined irrevocably with age (Woods 1996). The findings fitted the negative stereotypes of elderly people prevalent in western societies and were further supported by research indicating that the speed of neural transmissions in the central nervous system slowed with age (Botwinick 1977). This led to the assumption that the found cognitive deficits were due to an inevitable slowing of the brain's ability to process information (Birren and Schaie 1985). However, whilst this view appeared to have *ecological validity*, a different picture began to emerge when researchers probed more deeply into the relationship between ageing and cognitive decline.

First, it emerged that at least some of the decline in intelligence found with increasing age was attributable to *cohort effects* or generational differences in levels of education and prior exposure to IQ tests (Woods 1996). Second, researchers began to question, more generally, the assumption that intellectual ability was fixed at birth and irrevocably tied to the speed at which the brain could process information. Sternberg (1985), for example, argued that the intelligence tests on which such conclusions were based were inadequate measures of general intelligence, because they measured only intellectual, or academic, ability of the type taught in school, and took little account of factors such as the ability to profit and learn from experience and the ability to adapt successfully to a changing world. In line with this train of thought, it was argued that there was no reason why intelligence should not *increase* with age, as a function of continued learning and experience (Woods 1996). This position was further supported by developmental studies of children which showed that raw or innate intellectual ability could be boosted by the acquisition of learning strategies (Bee 1997).

The view that intelligence is not fixed at birth or defined exclusively by intellectual ability and speed of processing is broadly supported by Cattel's theory of intelligence, which posits that intelligence is composed of not one, but two, basic components, which are termed: *fluid intelligence* and *crystallised intelligence* (Horn and Cattel 1966). According to this theory, fluid intelligence is the fixed, inherited component of intelligence that determines the upper limits of the individual's ability to deal successfully with problems (particularly novel ones). This component *is* linked to the speed at which the brain processes information, and research has shown that it *does* decline with age (Hamilton 1996). Crystallised intelligence, on the other hand, represents the accumulation, or crystallisation, of learning through personal experience and the development of learning strategies that increase the individual's problem-solving abilities. Importantly, *this* component of intelligence appears to *increase* with age, provided that the individual remains stimulated and motivated to learn (Horn and Donaldson 1976). Indeed, Kimmel (1990) states that elderly people are as capable of learning new tricks (such as a second language) as their younger counterparts, but it takes them longer to do so (presumably because the information is processed more slowly).

In summing this up, a number of important inferences can be drawn. First, there is no a priori reason to believe that the elderly's ability to cope with challenging events should, on balance, be any worse than that of their younger counterparts, because they are likely to have an extensive range of coping responses in their repertoire, owing to their breadth of life experience. However, they are likely to deal with *novel situations* more slowly than their younger counterparts, and this should be borne in mind when, for example, admitting elderly people to hospital for the first time or when requiring them to master complicated self-care techniques at home.

Personality and age

I suggested earlier that the elderly's traits are typically painted in a negative light, and we may add that implicit in such perceptions is the assumption that they have not always been that way and the culprit is old age. However, contrary to popular belief, research has shown that personality remains relatively stable with increasing age and that the only reliable changes to occur are a shift towards an *external locus of control* (Lachman 1986) and a general shift towards *conservatism* and *rigidity* (Kermis 1984).

Let us ask what this might actually mean. Well, first, it is easy to envisage why a series of negative life events, such as the loss of one's spouse or experiencing a serious illness, might lead to a shift towards an external locus of control in the elderly person, who may come to believe that he or she has little direct control over their life. However, this can also happen to adults of all ages, so it is not an effect of ageing *per se*. Second, we might well define the shift towards rigidity as a general reluctance to break old habits and try new and innovative ways of dealing with events. However, we would have to concede that what may appear to be mere stubbornness could equally be viewed as simple preference for employing tried and tested coping mechanisms, which, by definition, are likely to be effective in the situations for which they are chosen. Nevertheless, it is conceivable that such rigidity might occasionally lead to a reluctance to try out new ways of dealing with problems, which in the worst case scenario could result in adherence to strategies that are inappropriate and detrimental to the self or others. This said, it is useful to view adherence to tried and tested coping responses as a mechanism by which the elderly may retain a sense of control and familiarity, and we should always take this into account when making judgements about the appropriateness of the individual's behaviour.

Ageing and coping

Self-efficacy, or the individual's beliefs about his or her ability to deal successfully with problems, may be heavily influenced by others' expectations. Rosenthal and Jacobsen (1968), for example, showed that a group of school children's overall academic performance was significantly enhanced after teachers had been inaccurately informed that they were 'high achievers'. Applying the reverse logic, researchers such as

Hayslip and Panek (1993) have been quick to point out that ageist stereotypes may result in correspondingly negative self-expectations in elderly people.

Kimmel (1990) suggests that elderly people often combat these effects by relying on an inherent sense of self-worth or self-esteem. However, it is not difficult to envisage how certain life events, such as a loss of status following retirement or a negative change in body image or personal abilities, may lower self-esteem, particularly when combined with the cumulative effects of negative stereotyping. Imagine, for example, an elderly man with cancer that necessitates surgical resection of the bowel and the permanent use of a colostomy bag. If, in learning to use the bag, he is inadvertently made to feel stupid and old by impatient care staff, his sense of self-worth and self-efficacy is likely to be severely impaired, leading to possible anger and depression.

Of course, difficulty in learning new self-care techniques is not confined to elderly patients, but there is a greater likelihood that decrements in this population will be attributed to internal characteristics (for instance, that of being old and cognitively impaired, etc.) than in a younger population, where external factors such as confusion caused by medication or anaesthesia are more likely to be considered. To an extent this is understandable. As we have learnt, elderly people *do* take longer to learn novel tasks, but there is another element at work too: Davies (1996) points out that nurses are most likely to have contact with elderly people who are ill, so there may be a tendency to overestimate the occurrence of negative events in old age.

Despite the latter author's appropriate caution, it does seem likely that the elderly's shift towards an external locus of control is, at least in part, a response to the cumulative effects of negative events and a feeling that life is beginning to take control of the self, rather than the reverse way round.

Kahana and Kahana (1982) argue that psychological well-being in old age is a function of the extent to which the elderly person's environment matches his or her personal needs. For example, a loss of perceived control is less likely to occur following the onset of disability if an individual with low dependency needs is subsequently placed in an environment designed to maximise his or her potential. By the same token, placing an individual with high dependency needs in an environment meant for autonomous individuals is only likely to remind the individual of what they are unable to do.

Ageing and physical decline

The majority of elderly people do *not* suffer from physical disorders that have a substantial effect on their ability to live their lives normally (Bromley 1988). However, they are more likely to be subject to a range of physical disorders that can impair cognitive processes and the ability to cope. Schaie (1990), for example, showed that even mild cardio-vascular disease can impair overall cognitive ability, and it is known that conditions affecting the body's metabolism, such as diabetes, de-hydration and constipation, can result in altered states of consciousness and confusion (Lancaster 1984).

Whilst confusional states can occur in any population, the elderly are particularly susceptible to causal imbalances in metabolism. For this reason, any marked and rapid alteration in cognitive ability should always be viewed as suggestive of some acute dysfunctional state that will impair the individual's ability to cope.

Summary

There is no convincing evidence that cognitive ability deteriorates as a function of age. Nor is there any substance in the belief that adverse changes in personality are irrevocably part and parcel of the ageing process. Rather, changes in cognitive ability and personality are largely a function of situational factors, such as physical illness, and stressful events, such as bereavement.

This may be summarised by *vulnerability* rather than *inevitability*. The elderly are vulnerable because of the effects of negative stereo-typing; they are vulnerable to the cumulative effects of stressful events and they are vulnerable to a range of physical conditions that may alter the body's metabolism. A decline in the elderly's ability to cope should not, therefore, be regarded as an inevitable function of age.

Summary

Depression is a relatively common condition that spans a continuum of disturbance ranging from episodes that are mild and transient to those that are severe, recurrent and resistant to treatment. There are two basic categories of depression: reactive and endogenous. According to the reactive view, depression is a response to adverse life events that may instil a sense of loss or learned helplessness. According to the endogenous view, however, the phenomenon of depression may be explained as a by-product of metabolic disturbance or imbalance.

Depression in hospital- and community-based populations often goes undetected and untreated, and in part this may be because nurses and other health professionals expect patients and their relatives to be emotionally upset following adverse events. Detecting depression requires good observation skills and a knowledge of the core symptoms, which include apathy, loss of libido, impaired cognitive functioning, feelings of guilt and low self-worth and repeated ideas of death and suicide. Normally, the presence of several of these features would be necessary for a formal diagnosis of depression.

There are four basic categories of theory that seek to explain the onset and maintenance of depression, and these include the faulty thinking model, the life events model, attachment theory and the biological model.

Chapter 9

Dying, bereavement and loss

Learning outcomes

By the end of this chapter you should be able to:

- Describe the four basic emotions associated with anticipated and actual loss.
- Outline the basic stages associated with the Kubler-Ross and Parkes models.
- Describe the pros and cons of stage models in clinical practice.

Dying, bereavement and loss: basic concepts

It is simple enough to define bereavement as a reaction occurring in response to the loss of someone or something close to us. However, in order to understand the nature of bereavement and the emotions and behaviours associated with it, it is important to ask *why* loss often affects people in such a devastating way. In answering this, we will start by examining the emotions most commonly experienced when a significant loss is anticipated or has actually occurred.

Emotional reactions to anticipated or actual loss

The anticipated loss of someone or something close to us, the loss of a body part or a loss of status are all threats to the self that can result in a sense of acute vulnerability. Such threats typically evoke a range of emotions, which include *fear* and *anger* (see Table 9.1). These emotions are considered to be primary in evolutionary terms, because when faced with a physical threat, fear motivated primitive man to run away and anger incited an aggressive response designed to ward off the threat (Berkowitz 1993).

Fear can arise for a variety of reasons, but it typically occurs in response to novel or previously unencountered events that threaten individuals in physical terms or which hold the perceived potential for outstripping their ability to cope. This fear of the unknown is often reflected in the concerns of dying patients, who report that the prospect of *losing control* can cause greater anxiety than the thought of dying *per se*. For example, patients often fear being unable to control basic bodily functions such as elimination, or fear losing control of their mental faculties, or experiencing uncontrollable pain (Carr 1982). Hence, fear is often *anticipatory* in nature and is arguably maladaptive, because, unlike primitive man faced with a physical threat, a dying patient cannot avoid the stressor by simply running away from it

TABLE 9.1 The four basic emotions associated with reactions to anticipated and actual loss

Emotion	Cause	Response
Fear	A sense of vulnerability	Motivation to avoid the stressor
Anger	A sense of frustration and a belief that others are to blame	Motivation to blame or hurt others
Guilt	A belief that one's actions have resulted in harm to another	Self-blame
Sadness	Severance of attachment and loss of an important part of the self	Intense grief and feelings of emptiness

(though they may, of course, employ defence mechanisms such as denial instead).

Anger, on the other hand, can be a positive force, as it can provide dying patients with the drive to overcome difficulties. Of course, anger can also be maladaptive and destructive, especially when vented as aggression towards members of family or staff. Although not condonable, such hostile reactions are understandable when one considers that anger and aggression are emotional responses that generally stem from intense *personal frustration* and the blocking of personal goals (Berkowitz 1993). There may be another element involved, however, because as Weiner (1986) points out, anger and aggression often stem from a sense of injustice and a belief that others are to blame. In fact, the tendency to apportion blame when misfortune strikes is common and appears to reflect a fundamental human need to find an explanation for untoward events.

To explain why this notion has clinical utility, we will borrow from Lerner's *belief in a just world* theory. Lerner (1975) proposes that people hold a belief in a just world, where the 'good guys' are rewarded and the 'bad guys' always get their just deserts. So when terminal illness, bereavement or some other catastrophic event strikes, the individual is driven to explain why the world has not operated in a just and fair way. Imagine, for example, a mother that has just lost a small child as a consequence of leukaemia. According to her belief system, such things don't simply 'happen', so she seeks a reason for her loss by attributing blame either to herself ('it was my fault . . . if only I'd sought help earlier') or to others ('it was the doctor's fault . . . he misdiagnosed the symptoms'). Either way, she is likely to feel considerable anger towards herself or towards the care staff.

Although this might sound like an undesirable and maladaptive response, we should consider what might happen if she was unable to attribute blame for her child's death to some internal or external source. In answer to this, it seems likely that she would be forced to abandon her belief in a just world and pressed to adopt a new belief, which was based on the premise that the world is a dangerous place where untoward events occur at random and without reason. Hardly a comforting thought for someone struggling to come to terms with a major loss (incidentally, you may recall that this was exactly the type of belief thrust violently upon PTSD victims). In short, attributing blame internally or externally helps to maintain a psychological equilibrium by providing an explanation (which may or may not be illusory) that is not at odds with the individual's view of the world.

Whereas *fear* and *anger* are, arguably, the most powerful emotions associated with *anticipated loss*, a feeling of overwhelming *sadness* is the most pervasive emotional response to *actual loss* (Parkes 1972). The acute sadness or grief associated with loss or bereavement may be explained using a self-system framework similar to that outlined in Part One. According to this framework, things of value to us are incorporated into our self-system over time, until the person, animal, ideal or object becomes an integral 'part' of us (Cooley 1902). When that thing is lost, the individual's sense of self is violated and a vacuum is left that cannot immediately be filled. Bowlby (1969) explains this reaction in terms of the severance of an emotional attachment that has been important to the individual. Of course, we cannot see such processes happening directly, but bereaved people often report a deep sense of emptiness and a sense of loss that has an almost physical quality (Parkes and Weiss 1983).

The final emotion commonly associated with bereavement is guilt. According to Buss (1980), guilt typically occurs when individuals believe that their actions have resulted in harm to someone else. Indeed, it is not uncommon for bereaved persons to feel that they should have acted sooner, been more attentive or avoided saying something that leaves them with a feeling of regret and a sense of self-blame

(Parkes 1986). These attributions are normal and generally subside with the passage of time. However, intense and protracted feelings of guilt often indicate the presence of an *abnormal grief reaction* that may warrant professional help (Carr 1982).

Models of death and dying

There are two principal *stage models* that deal with the human reactions to loss and bereavement. The Kubler-Ross model (1969) details a stereotypical pattern of response that occurs when the individual anticipates death or the loss of a body part or some important body function, and Parkes (1986) highlights the typical bereavement reaction that occurs in response to the actual loss of someone close.

Despite the differences in focus, there is considerable overlap in each model's descriptions of the responses that occur to anticipated and actual loss.

The Kubler-Ross model

According to the Kubler-Ross model, an individual faced with the prospect of imminent death, or the loss of some important function, typically proceeds through five recognisable stages (see Table 9.2).

TABLE 9.2 The Kubler-Ross model of death and dying

Stage	Characteristics
1 Denial	Cushions the impact of reality
2 Anger	Results from sense of injustice and frustration
3 Bargaining	Attempts to negate or reduce the threat posed to the self by negotiation
4 Depression	The finality of death or loss is acknowledged and sense of helplessness or hopelessness is evoked
5 Acceptance	Death is accepted and the individual is at peace with the inevitable

The first stage involves *denial*, which arises when the individual finds it difficult to accept the reality of the situation. Hence, denial may be seen as a protective mechanism that grants the individual time to assimilate the full meaning of the event. The second stage involves *anger*, which stems from a feeling of injustice and frustration, as the significance of the event sinks home. During the third stage, the individual tries to strike a *bargain* (for example with medical staff or God) in an attempt to stave off the threat of death. At a cognitive or practical level, bargaining may result in the patient's decision to co-operate fully with treatment regimes in the hope that this may buy precious time. However, at an emotional level, it may result in regressive, child-like reactions, which are best dealt with by offering reassurance and emotional support.

During the fourth stage, the individual experiences *depression*, as it becomes clear to the patient that his or her efforts to change the situation are futile. The presence of depression may be taken to indicate that the individual has acknowledged the inevitability of death.

According to the model, the fifth and final stage is marked by an *acceptance* of the inevitable. The feelings of depression are eased and the individual is no longer terrified of dying. He or she is able to review their life and draw their personal affairs to a close in discussion with their loved ones.

Parkes' model of bereavement

Parkes (1986) suggests that bereaved individuals progress through four stages: numbness, pining, disorganisation and despair and recovery. Stage one is marked by a *numbness* or *denial* that may last for minutes, hours or days and occasionally weeks. As in the Kubler-Ross model, the individual has difficulty in accepting the reality of death and may appear dazed and unresponsive, or stoical and calm, proceeding as though nothing had happened (Carr 1981).

As the reality of the situation begins to hit home, the individual enters the second stage, which is characterised by *pining* or *yearning* for the deceased. The bereaved individual may instinctively *search* the house or neighbourhood to check that their loved one is not simply lost somewhere or hurt. This preoccupation with the deceased can also give rise to very real *illusions*, or false perceptions, that can be disturbing. For example, creaking floorboards may be interpreted as the deceased moving around the house. The smell of someone's perfume may lead to a visual search in a crowd, or a shadow in a corner may take the shape of his or her personage. Such events suggest that the attentional processes are flooded with thoughts and emotions about the deceased, perhaps in much the same way as can happen to individuals suffering from post traumatic stress disorder.

During this second stage, the bereaved person often has a strong need to talk with people who knew the deceased and may want to spend a great deal of time going over the circumstances surrounding his or her death. This process, which other people sometimes find uncomfortable and disconcerting, is sometimes referred to as *'reality testing'* and it appears to help the individual accept the finality of death. Indeed, it has been argued that the period of *mourning*, characterised by rituals such as the funeral and the wake, are traditions that have developed to help meet this need (Parkes and Weiss 1983). By the same token, it is often particularly hard for the bereaved person to comprehend the reality of death when there is no corpse or concrete evidence of death, as may occur, for example, when someone is missing and presumed dead, at sea or in combat (Wright 1986).

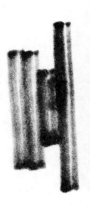

The third phase, which may last for several months, is marked by intense and acute feelings of *despair* and *depression*. As in the Kubler-Ross model, the reality of death is now accepted and the individual is forced to grapple with the full implications of the loss. This realisation catapults the individual into a turmoil of emotional, cognitive and behavioural disorganisation that is characterised by very high levels of arousal, acute despair and often anger (Parkes 1986). During this stage emotional and cognitive restructuring must take place. Janis (1958) referred to this as *worry work*, as it involves making sense of the death, coming to terms with future roles and *compartmentalising* the strong emotions that beset the individual. Only when this restructuring has been successfully achieved can the individual move forward.

Sometimes individuals get 'stuck' in this phase. This may, for example, occur when a bereaved mother is unable to make sense of the death of her child or is unable to reconcile her part in it. Such prolonged grief reactions, or *chronic sorrow*, are often marked by intense feelings of anger, in response to a sense of injustice and frustration, or feelings of guilt, in response to feelings of personal responsibility and a belief that the death could have been avoided (Weiss 1993).

During the fourth and final stage, which is one of *recovery* and *reorganisation*, the individual finds that they begin to become less

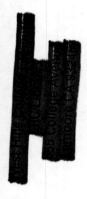

preoccupied with thoughts of the deceased. The individual's task is now to build a new self-identity and to move forward (Parkes 1972) (though Carr (1982) notes that elderly individuals may lack the motivation to do this). This stage often commences at around nine to twelve months and reflects the fact that the individual is beginning to work successfully though the loss. During this period, certain stimuli (such as hearing a 'favourite' piece of music or being aware of changes in the seasons) may retrigger memories, which can rekindle the feelings of intense grief present in stage three. Gradually, however, these episodes become less frequent and the individual begins to plan ahead, which is a sign that recovery is well under way. The stages just discussed are summarised in Table 9.3.

TABLE 9.3 A model of bereavement adapted from Parkes (1986) and Carr (1981)

Stage	Characteristics
Numbness or denial	A state of shock caused by the implications of death. A defence mechanism that cushions the self from reality
Yearning or pining	Searching behaviour and seeking confirmation of death or 'reality testing'
Despair or depression	Grappling with the finality of death. Emotional, cognitive and behavioural disorganisation and restructuring of the self
Recovery	Diminished preoccupation with the deceased. Begins to look forward and plan for the future

The pros and cons of stage models

Stage models provide a useful framework that can be used to make sense of the bewildering emotional and behavioural reactions that accompany dying and bereavement. They can help the nurse to stand back and view anger as a response to threat or the need to apportion blame, and they provide a rough guide to the processes involved in coming to terms with actual or anticipated loss. Their main drawback is that they may be accepted as rigid frameworks, with the accompanying expectation that the patient *should* progress through them in an orderly, sequential manner. In fact, individuals typically oscillate between stages. An individual in the recovery stage of bereavement may be catapulted back to the despair stage by some external, triggering cue. Alternatively, anger may be persistently used by a dying patient as a means of maintaining a sense of control, the loss of which might otherwise lead to depression and despair.

The Kubler-Ross model, in particular, can conjure up an over-simplified model of dying, where the patient receives an initial diagnosis that leads to a linear progression through the stages, which culminates neatly in acceptance. Yet, in reality, terminal illness often evokes a *series of crises*, which may be precipitated by events, such as surgery, having to give up work, loss of continence, being unable to maintain a sexual relationship, loss of mobility, an inability to digest food, etc. So the emotional turmoil created by the original diagnosis is often only one of a series of events that involve a pattern of crisis, adaptation, a plateau of relative calm, another crisis, adaptation and so on.

On a broader level, when thinking about patients with non-terminal, but serious or debilitating disease, we should be wary of the assumption that individuals typically reach a stage of acceptance, when it is probably more realistic to *expect* adaptation to loss in many instances (Russell 1993). Furthermore, as Shontz (1982) points out, adaptation is not necessarily equated with adopting the disabled role expected by society. For example, a teenager paralysed from the waist down in a road traffic accident may reject any notion of being crippled or different in any way and may subsequently engage in strenuous and demanding sporting activities to prove his or her case. Given this perspective, we should also think carefully about what we expect in terms of 'acceptance' in chronically and terminally ill patients.

Turning to one final issue, Wortman and Silva (1989) have challenged the widely held notion that individuals must experience a period of intense despair and depression if they are to avoid a delayed grief reaction and misery further down the road. In fact, these authors' trawl of the literature revealed wide-ranging variations in the extent to which individuals experienced acute grief and despair and only limited evidence connecting an absence of grief with later depression. So again we need to exercise caution in expecting 'typical' reactions.

Summing all of this up, we can assume only that reactions to actual or anticipated loss are complex and subject to individual differences. These differences mean that we should view stage models of death, dying and bereavement as potentially useful clinical tools, whilst avoiding the expectation that every patient will conform to a given stereotype. Furthermore, we also need to consider that the events associated with death and dying often evoke a series of crises that may *each* involve denial, anger, bargaining, etc. In fact, armed with this knowledge, it is probably better to try and avoid gauging which 'stage' the patient has entered and to focus instead on the context in which reactions occur and to ask the question 'Why is the patient reacting in this way?'

Summary

Individuals initially react to challenging events by appraising the extent of the physical or psychological threat that they face and then assessing whether or not they have the resources available to cope. These resources include social support, the individual's characteristic traits and habitual methods of dealing with challenging events. The effectiveness of such resources will be tempered by the individual's expectancies, which can be positive or negative, depending upon past experiences.

Occasionally, stressful events result in the development of phobic reactions, which are particularly likely to occur when the stressor is traumatic and the individual is vulnerable. When threats to the self cannot be avoided, the individual may seek to reduce the impact of the event by employing denial. Anger, and then sadness, eventually replaces denial as the primary emotion as reality is gradually absorbed. Guilt may also be experienced if the individual believes that his or her actions or failure to take action resulted in avoidable harm to their loved one. These emotions are normal and are usually transient. However, the existence of such intense feelings over a protracted period is often an indication that professional help may be required.

Kubler-Ross and Parkes describe a series of stages that patients may work through when loss is anticipated or has actually occurred. Taken together, the descriptions show how individuals may move from an initial state of denial, disbelief and disorganisation, through to a state of acceptance or adaptation that may be viewed as a rebuilding of the self and a constructive move forward.

1   Describe the basic processes involved in primary and secondary appraisal.

2   Explain why factors such as social support, self-esteem support and instrumental support may help the individual to deal with stressful events.

3   What conditions are likely to evoke a state of learned helplessness?

4   Describe the defining features of a phobia.

5   Briefly explain how conditioned responses, such as anticipatory nausea, may be avoided using basic nursing interventions.

6   Describe the main features of post traumatic stress disorder.

7   Explain why aggression is more likely to occur in stressful situations.

8   Outline the four principal causes of depression.

9   Describe the four main emotional responses associated with loss reactions.

10 In what ways are stage models potentially misleading?

REFLECTIVE SCENARIOS

Annalisa

Annalisa is 42 years of age and twenty weeks pregnant. A test has shown that her baby has Down's Syndrome and she and her husband are both feeling very stressed.

Explore their reaction with reference to threat appraisal and discuss the broad, psycho-social factors that may mediate their response.

Sanjay

Sanjay is a self-employed construction worker, who has been unable to find work for several months. He is married with two children and has a large financial commitment on his house. He has tried to find alternative forms of work without success and has taken to drinking excessively during the day. This has only added to the financial pressures he faces, and his actions have palpably raised the stress levels of every family member.

Using the crisis model detailed in Part two, explain what may happen if Sanjay is unable to find a satisfactory solution to his problems.

Tom

Tom is a 3 year old whose weight lies around the tenth centile, despite both his parents' weight and height being above the norm. He was born with a severe cleft palate, which necessitated tube-feeding for the first nine months of life. The deformity has since been surgically corrected so that he is able to chew and swallow solids, but he vomits whenever he is presented with any kind of food with lumps in it.

Explain the possible reasons for his behaviour using a classical conditioning framework.

Sarah

You may recall from Part One that Sarah gave birth to a premature boy by emergency caesarean section. The events surrounding this were traumatic. She had gone to the maternity unit for a routine check-up and ended up being rushed to theatre at top speed with little explanation or time for preparation. Six weeks have now elapsed since her discharge from the maternity unit and her son is doing well. However, Sarah's mood is unstable. Her sleep is often punctuated by nightmares, she feels anxious and depressed and is unable to stop fantasising negatively about what may have happened to her son in the operating theatre.

Explain the possible reasons for Sarah's condition with reference to stress appraisal and post traumatic stress disorder.

Bill

Bill is a 23-year-old male with learning difficulties and a history of violent behaviour towards care staff. He has recently been admitted to an acute psychiatric ward following detention by the police. The staff at the unit do not particularly want him there. They feel he is a social services case and twice in three days he is prepared for discharge, which is cancelled each time.

Given these circumstances, discuss the psychological factors that increase the risk of another violent assault on a member of staff.

Sanphy

Sanphy is a second year student nurse who has just been verbally ravaged by Rebecca, a middle-aged woman who is being treated for inoperable cancer of the liver. You witnessed the event and feel you need to talk to Sanphy about the reasons for Rebecca's outburst.

Explain how you might do this with special reference to the Kubler-Ross model and your knowledge of the causes of anger and aggression.

Eunice

Eunice is a 64-year-old woman who has recently suffered a cerebral stroke, resulting in marked aphasia and some loss of mobility. Her daughter is concerned about her and tells you that Eunice has been quite weepy following the stroke and does not seem like her normal self. *Explain what you might do to explore whether or not Eunice is depressed.*

Diane

Diane recently lost her daughter and husband in a horrific car accident involving a drunken driver. The experience was harrowing: she was called to formally identify their bodies and endured a public hearing where the coroner read explicit details of their injuries and mode of death. Diane has been unable to move their belongings since the tragedy and frequently experiences intense feelings of guilt and hatred. *With reference to Parkes' model of bereavement, discuss the extent to which her reaction lies within normal boundaries.*

Suggested reading

Johnston, M. and Wallace, L. (1990). *Stress and Medical Procedures.* Oxford: Oxford University Press.
This book provides useful information about the factors contributing to patient stress in medicine, surgery, obstetrics and paediatric care.

Joseph, S., Williams, R. and Yule, W. (1997). *Understanding Post-Traumatic Stress: A psychosocial perspective.* Chichester: JohnWiley and Sons.
This recent text is well written and provides a comprehensive overview of PTSD.

Marks, I. M. (1997). *Living With Fear: Understanding and coping with anxiety.* Maidenhead: McGraw Hill.
This reprint of the 1978 version provides a wide-ranging and informative account of the nature of anxiety and anxiety disorders, together with a lucid account of behavioural treatments for phobias and aversive reactions.

Parkes, C. M. (1986). *Bereavement: Studies of grief in adult life.* 6th ed. London: Tavistock.
This is the latest version of this classic text on bereavement.

Woods, T. (Ed.) (1996). *Handbook of Clinical Psychology of Ageing*. Beckenham: Crook-Helm.
This book provides a comprehensive overview of current psychological research into psycho-social issues and ageing.

Part three

Promoting
and maintaining
health

Chapter 10

Health protective
behaviour

Learning outcomes

By the end of this chapter you should be able to:

- Outline the main psychological factors associated with the detection of signs and symptoms of illness.
- Outline the health belief model and the theory of reasoned action.
- Describe how stress may affect decision-making.

This section deals with two main topics, the first of which provides an overview of the factors that have been shown to influence *help-seeking behaviour*, or people's decisions to seek professional help for signs and symptoms of illness. This is an issue of considerable importance, because failure to seek help at an early stage can lead to an unnecessary worsening of the patient's condition and, in some cases, premature death.

The second topic deals with the phenomenon of *non-compliance* with nursing and medical advice, which, it has been estimated, may be responsible for as many as one in five admissions to hospital (Ley 1982).

In the following discussion, the term *health protective behaviour* will be used to refer to the concepts of help-seeking behaviour and compliance and non-compliance.

Help-seeking behaviour

The early detection of symptoms has long been recognised as a key factor in the fight against disease and has figured prominently in health education campaigns designed to help people to recognise somatic changes that might signal the onset of conditions, such as cancer and meningitis. Such campaigns are often directed at vulnerable target groups, based upon characteristics such as age, gender, ethnicity, social class, genetic risk and behavioural habits, and are designed to foster attentive or *vigilant behaviour* that will prompt early help-seeking behaviour.

Symptom detection, however, is a relatively complex process. The early symptoms of disease may be benign or may overlap with more common, and less serious, conditions. Added to this, the individual brings his or her own experiences, expectations and beliefs to the fore, which can result in widely differing interpretations of similar somatic cues. Also, emotional states, such as fear and anxiety, can give rise to selective inattention or denial of presenting symptoms. In short, individual differences play an important role in the process of symptom detection, and before a decision is made to seek professional advice for suspected illness the individual must:

- Be attentive to the presence of internal, somatic stimuli.
- Interpret the stimuli as potential symptoms of illness.

Given that these interdependent factors underpin symptom detection, we will now explore each in a little more detail.

Detection of symptoms

In the hustle and bustle of modern life, people are bombarded with a wide range of stimuli, and innocuous symptoms of illness may easily go undetected. However, our attention is most likely to be drawn to symptoms that involve *pain* or *discomfort*, or which affect our ability to *function* normally, or which stand out because they are perceived to be unusual or *abnormal* in some way. Similarly, individuals who believe that they are at an increased risk, or are *vulnerable* to certain forms of physical or psychological illness, are likely to be particularly vigilant, or 'on the look out', for associated signs and symptoms (Becker and Rosenstock 1984).

Symptom detection, however, is also affected by emotional states, which may result in a decrease *or* increase in the likelihood of help-seeking behaviour. For example, anxiety can lead to selective inattention or denial of symptoms, but can also lead to a state of *hypervigilance*, where the individual becomes overly sensitive to internal feedback from the body's systems, leading to the misinterpretation of normal physiological responses as signs of illness or dysfunction (Steptoe and Mathews 1984). In extreme cases, this may take the form of *hypochondriasis*, where the individual is constantly focused on internal, somatic stimuli and is consumed by concern about some underlying pathology. When this concern is centred on a single condition, it is labelled an *illness phobia* (Marks 1997).

In summing this up, we can state that symptom detection is dependent upon the:

- Strength of the underlying symptoms, including features such as pain, discomfort, unusualness and embarrassment.

- Degree of competing stimuli in the individual's environment.
- Individual's emotional state.
- Individual's sense of vulnerability.

Perception of symptoms

Our perception of symptoms and what they might mean is largely dependent upon our prior levels of knowledge and experience. Furthermore, research has shown that we have 'common sense' models of illness that contain beliefs about the causes and consequences of symptoms and which subsequently guide our decisions to seek (or not to seek) professional help from a medical practitioner or a nurse (Lau and Hartman 1983; Meyer *et al.* 1985). For the sake of continuity, we will refer to these models as *illness schemas* that influence the detection and perception of symptoms. For example, you would probably have little trouble listing the common symptoms of influenza, together with an estimate of how long you would expect the symptoms to last; should the symptoms become unusual or particularly severe, or if they persisted beyond your expectations, the chances are you would be motivated to seek professional help.

These illness schemas appear to be quite effective, as the proportion of people seeking medical help for symptoms of common illness is generally very low, varying between 7 per cent and 26 per cent (Pitts 1991). Research has also shown that when people are concerned about unusual, abnormal or persistent symptoms, they typically discuss them with a confidant, such as a friend, spouse, colleague, priest, etc., before seeking professional help (Zola 1973). Indeed, Scrambler and Scrambler (1984) found that eleven 'lay consultations' took place for every medical consultation. This *lay-referral system* has been highlighted as important by a number of researchers, because medical help is typically sought only after a confidant has advised that, in their view, the symptoms are unusual and warrant further investigation (Zola 1973). Of course, the system may fail when symptoms warranting urgent help are misinterpreted as benign through ignorance or lack of knowledge.

Individuals are also reluctant to confide in others when the location and nature of the symptoms cause embarrassment (such as may occur with rectal or vaginal problems) or when the symptoms may be attributed to some condition that carries a social stigma (such as may occur with sexually transmitted disease). In short, the presence of certain symptoms may actually inhibit help-seeking behaviour (Becker and Rosenstock 1984).

This barrier also appears to operate when mental health problems are involved. For example, unpublished research undertaken by myself and a colleague investigating first-time contacts with a Community Mental Health Service in South Devon, revealed that clients with mental health problems typically waited several months before approaching their general practitioner (GP) for referral. When asked whether they had confided in someone prior to approaching their GP, they revealed that they had found it difficult to confide in other people, because they believed that others lacked knowledge of mental health problems and were concerned about being perceived as insane (Russell and Towler 1990). Thus, the lay-referral system had apparently failed, because *norms* for signs and symptoms of conditions, such as depression, anxiety and psychosis, were lacking or totally absent. Indeed, the investigation revealed that it was often a resulting crisis that eventually led individuals to seek professional help, and these findings have been echoed by Clausen and Radke Yarrow (1995) investigating hospitalisation for individuals with schizophrenia.

Cultural influences may also affect the individual's perception of illness, and in some societies illness may be perceived as a consequence of supernatural forces, such as witchcraft, rather than by a viral or bacterial agent for which they have no concept. For example, a sudden event such as paralysis might logically be blamed on some invading evil spirit by people that have no awareness of causal factors such as poliomyelitis or intracranial bleeding.

Age is a further factor that has an important influence on the individual's perception of illness. For example, elderly people may simply *misattribute* signs and symptoms of disease to 'old age' and accordingly fail to seek help (Janz and Becker 1984). Similarly, a pregnant working mother may attribute symptoms such as frequent headaches and swollen ankles to stress, rather than perceiving them as a possible symptom of problems with her pregnancy.

At the opposite end of the spectrum, the young child's illness schema is much less sophisticated than that of an adult, and they generally perceive the causes and consequences of illness in relatively simple terms. Pre-school children, for example, tend to view all forms of illness as contagious. Thus, they may believe that heart disease can be 'caught' by standing next to someone. If you think about this, it is quite a logical belief, as most of the common illnesses the youngster will have experienced will be of a contagious nature (i.e. colds, measles, chicken-pox, head lice, etc.). Similarly, young children sometimes view illness as punishment for having been naughty, and they are generally unable to perceive the causes of major illnesses as mutifactorial until they near their teens (Bibbace and Walsh 1980). (The exceptions to this rule may occur in children who have direct, personal experience of a major illness, such as diabetes, haemophilia, etc. In such circumstances, their illness schemas can be very sophisticated.)

Finally, gender can also play a significant role in the perception of illness and is linked to our expectations about the relative probability of contracting some disease or illness. For example, people know that certain illnesses tend to be (or are) gender-specific, and therefore males and females are likely to be differentially vigilant in detecting signs and symptoms of illness related to gender-specific conditions. If, for example, you are a 50-year-old male and a heavy smoker, you are unlikely to be concerned about breast cancer and are more likely to be vigilantly aware of the symptoms of heart or lung disease.

In summarising what we have learnt so far, we can state that perception of illness (and help-seeking behaviour) is influenced by:

- Personal knowledge and experience.
- The lay-referral system.
- Stigma and embarrassment.
- Cultural influences.
- Age.
- Gender.

Models of health behaviour

The health belief model

During the past twenty years, a number of theoretical models have been constructed to explain individual differences in health protective behaviour. Of these models, the first (and still the most widely referred to) is the *health belief model* (HBM), which was devised in the late 1960s by Rosenstock and subsequently modified by co-researchers Janz and Becker in 1984. The model is uncomplicated and its intuitive appeal has led to its common application in two important areas of primary health care, where emphasis is placed upon:

- Encouraging people to seek early professional help for signs and symptoms of illness.
- Improving uptake on preventative health programmes such as immunisation and screening for disease.

According to the model, health protective behaviours, such as the decision to seek professional help, are influenced by a relatively small number of factors (see Figure 10.1). For example, the likelihood of taking preventative action is increased when the individual has a sense of *perceived vulnerability*. This may occur when he or she believes that their symptoms are indicative of something severe or when there is a family history that renders them susceptible to certain conditions. Any perception of vulnerability is further mediated by variables such as age, sex and the individual's prior beliefs. So, a male in his early twenties, with a strong history of family heart disease, may be lulled into a false sense of security, because he knows that heart disease typically affects middle-aged males.

The model also predicts that the likelihood of engaging in health protective behaviour is influenced by the perceived *costs versus benefits* of taking a particular course of action (Becker and Rosenstock 1984). Imagine, for example, that you are a parent considering whether to have your 15-month-old child immunised against measles, mumps and

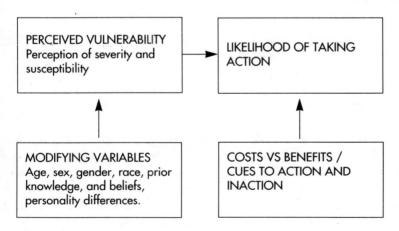

FIGURE 10.1 The health belief model

rubella (MMR). In making the decision, you might weigh up the potential benefits (i.e. reduced risk of severe infection with secondary complications, less time away from school, etc.) against the potential costs (i.e. subjecting your child to pain, the possibility of side effects and subsequent complications, etc.). Similarly, someone deciding whether or not to have major surgery and radiotherapy for advanced cancer may decide that the probability of a cure is low, whilst the likelihood of pain and discomfort resulting from treatment is high.

Finally, the model suggests that certain stimuli may function as *cues to action*, increasing the likelihood of engaging in protective behaviours, whilst others may function as *barriers to action*, decreasing the likelihood. These cues commonly include:

Cues to action that increase the likelihood of health protective behaviour

- Health promotion campaigns.
- Lay-referral system.
- Pain and personal discomfort.
- Pressure to take action emanating from third parties, such as the individual's spouse, friends, employer, etc.

Cues to inaction that decrease the likelihood of health protective behaviour

- Innocuous symptoms.
- Denial/avoidance of anxiety.
- Negative health promotion campaigns.
- Personal or social crises (such as divorce and bereavement).
- Stigma inherent in seeking help for certain conditions.

It should be noted that, although media campaigns may successfully promote health protective behaviours, they may also induce avoidance of the issue they seek to address (Sarrafino 1994). This is most likely to occur when the campaigning is negative (i.e. induces fear) or when individuals believe that they would be unable to change their behaviour (such as with an addiction to nicotine or alcohol)

Problems with the HBM

The HBM provides the health professional with a good model with which to understand health protective behaviours. Like all models, however, it does not allow 100 per cent prediction of behaviour (Janz and Becker 1984).

The reasons for this are quite straightforward. First, the model is most likely to tell us something about the probable health behaviours of a *general target group*, or population of people. For example, we might correctly predict that those most likely to engage in testicular self-examination for cancer would be males who perceived themselves to be vulnerable (i.e. had a family history) and who were in the highest risk age group (typically 20–30). However, the model would be less useful when making predictions about behaviour at the *level of the individual*, because of the effect of modifying variables, such as personal beliefs, traits, prior experiences and idiosyncratic or habitual behaviour. For example, a male might hold the superstitious belief that focusing on testicular cancer makes it more likely to happen, or he might have a fatalistic personality trait (Reed *et al.* 1994) which leads him to believe that he has little or no personal control over disease processes or outcomes. Furthermore, a history of adverse experiences can result in anxiety, denial and avoidance of professional help. For example, Antonovosky and Hartman (1974) found that some women stopped carrying out breast self-examination after a number of *false-positives* led to periods of high anxiety.

These issues aside, Janz and Becker (1984) argue that the HBM does allow reasonably accurate prediction of a wide range of health protective behaviours, and, despite the tabled limitations, it does provide a framework for understanding the individual patient's behaviour.

Other 'models' include *protection motivation* theory and the *health action* process, the interested reader is encouraged to refer to texts such as Sarrafino (1994) and Bennet and Murphy (1997).

The theory of reasoned action

According to the *theory of reasoned action* (TRA), the individual's stated *intention* to perform a certain act is an important factor in predicting behaviour (Ajzen and Fishbein 1980). Whilst this may not sound like a particularly earth-shattering find, the authors argue that a knowledge of someone's intentions provides more accurate information than that afforded by knowing what someone's *attitude* is towards a certain thing or course of action.

In order to understand why this should be, we need to examine briefly the nature of attitudes. In fact, an attitude is quite a complex phenomenon that comprises an *affective component* (the way we feel about things), a *cognitive component* (our beliefs and expectations) and a *behavioural component* (how these feelings and cognitions are translated into actual behaviour) (Atkinson *et al.* 1993). In consideration of this, the point to note is that there is often a less than perfect correlation between the affective and cognitive components and actual behaviour. Imagine, for example, that a young student nurse is approached by a health psychologist who is carrying out an investigation into attitudes towards bone-marrow donation. The student is asked a series of questions such as, 'Do you think that bone-marrow transplant procedures should be fully funded by the NHS?', and 'Would you be in favour of establishing a national register of potential donors?' No doubt the student would reply yes to both questions and, in doing so, would have expressed a positive attitude towards bone-marrow transplants. However, we might be less confident that the student would actually offer him or herself as a donor if subsequently asked to do so. In short, attitudes are often a poor predictor of behaviour, because they sometimes sample what people feel they *ought to do,*

The TRA attempts to make some allowance for this difficulty by sampling the individual's *personal attitudes*, stated *intentions* and the *normative attitudes* held by others, such as family, friends, neighbours, etc. (see Figure 10.2). In doing so, the TRA makes some allowance for so-called *social facilitation effects*, or the extent to which an individual's behaviour is likely to be influenced by others' attitudes and behaviours. It is quite easy to conceptualise this in practice. Say, for example, that a community-based midwife is interested in promoting breast-feeding in a first-time mother-to-be and spends quite a bit of time providing her with positive information. Persuaded, the woman tells the midwife that she intends to breast feed, because she believes it will be beneficial to her baby. However, although ever hopeful, the midwife is less convinced that this positive attitude will actually be translated into behaviour, because she knows that most of the local mothers bottle-feed and hold quite negative attitudes towards breast-feeding. Accordingly, even if the mother-to-be's stated intention is more than a mere social

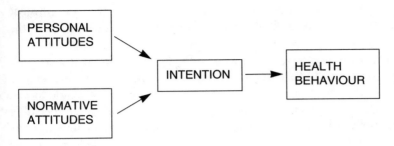

FIGURE 10.2 The theory of reasoned action

facilitation effect, the pressures that will be brought to bear on her will be considerable. (In consideration of this point, you might like to think about how many barriers are presented to women who want to breast feed in a society, neighbourhood or family that is non-supportive.) The underlying message here is that it is important to target communities, as well as the individual, when promoting health protective behaviours.

Problems with the TRA

One of the criticisms levelled at the TRA is that it takes no account of the extent to which individuals believe that they can execute a desired behaviour. For example, we might have reason to believe that an individual high in self-efficacy would be more likely to carry out an intention to engage in health protective behaviour than an individual low in self-efficacy and lacking in self-confidence. For this reason, Ajzen (1985) modified the TRA by adding the component *perceived control*, and renaming the theory: the *theory of reasoned action* and planned behaviour.

Making health decisions under conditions of stress

A criticism that is sometimes targeted at the HBM, TRA and like models is that they adopt the premise that health protective behaviour is guided by rational decision-making, which creates an illusion of scientific precision (Steptoe and Mathews 1984; Leventhal *et al.* 1997).

There is, however, a considerable body of research that indicates that this basic premise is fallible. For example, you may recall that the Yerkes-Dodson Law predicts that high levels of anxiety affect our ability to think clearly. So it is not difficult to imagine that a couple's judgement would be more subject to the effects of stress and anxiety when having to decide whether or not to terminate a 20-week-old foetus, because of a potentially serious abnormality, than when deciding whether or not to have their first child immunised. Some investigators have argued that high levels of anxiety can cloud judgement and impede rational decision-making under conditions of stress, because the individual's state of mind is fundamentally altered.

These different states of mind have been characterised by the terms *hot* and *cold cognitions* (Janis and Mann 1979; Zaborowski and Oleszkiewicz 1988). Cold cognitions are associated with logical decision-making processes that are essentially neutral in emotional or affective terms, whereas hot cognitions are associated with decision-making processes that are laden with affect, such as high levels of anxiety or low self-esteem and depression. In fact, if we relate this to our knowledge of the self-system, we might argue that hot cognitions are essentially those that occur when some aspect or component of the self is threatened.

According to Janis and Mann's *conflict theory* (1979), individuals faced with a life-threatening crisis often think irrationally and their ability to make the best possible decision is compromised. Indeed, the authors argue that rational decision-making can take place *only* when the individual a) believes that there are alternative courses of action available, b) has sufficient information to make an informed choice and c) believes that there is adequate time available to act upon one of the alternatives. Without the presence of these three conditions, the individual is likely to adopt one of the following courses of action:

- Panic and accept the first available solution.
- Deny the gravity of events and behave as though nothing untoward has happened.
- Divert attention to other things and/or shift responsibility for the event onto others.

These reactions, which represent panic, denial and avoidance respectively, may also be linked to a perceived loss of control, which may well be alleviated by providing the patient with information about possible alternatives. So, as well as providing information about the probable outcomes of surgery – the risks, possible complications, pain, side effects, etc. – we might also seek to provide the patient with information about natural death, the likely time-span, the likelihood of pain and available pain relief, possible hospice or home care, etc.

Finally, circumstances may occasionally arise (such as in terminal illness) where individuals simply do not want to discuss their condition or consider further the options that might be available to them. In such instances, it is important to respect the patient's decision, unless you have strong grounds to believe that his or her actions are founded on a lack of information or misconception.

Focus on clinical practice: quality of life

Quality of life (QOL) is an important concept that has proved difficult to define, because it has many meanings. At a general level, the term conjures an image of how happy or satisfied the individual is with his or her lot. However, Draper (1997) states that its meaning may vary depending on whether it is used as an *objective measure* to evaluate and generate social policy and make decisions about how to allocate scarce resources, or whether it is used as a *subjective measure* to evaluate the effects of nursing practice or medical treatments at the level of the individual. For most nurses, it is the latter aspect of QOL that is particularly salient.

In order to understand the meaning of QOL, Draper (1997) suggests that we need to step back and reflect upon a) what it means to be human and b) under what conditions humans typically thrive. In consideration of this, he argues that when evaluating QOL we should turn our attention to basic concepts such as *dignity, autonomy, choice, privacy* and *self-development,* and to this we may add *relief from pain and discomfort, hopelessness* and *self-condemnation* (Johal 1995).

According to Eiser (1994) and Johal (1995), there has been a tendency in medical practice to view extension of life as sufficient grounds for the implementation of aggressive medical interventions without sufficient consideration of the effects on the individual's overall QOL. Such concerns, however, extend beyond the realms of nursing in general medical settings and into wider fields of nursing practice, such as child nursing, learning disabilities and mental health (Wright 1994; Smith 1995; Collier 1997).

QOL and learning disabilities

During the 1960s and 1970s, health professionals became increasingly concerned about the effects of *institutionalisation* on patients living in large institutions. Following the work of investigators such as Goffman (1961) and Szasz (1975), institutionalisation became synonymous with depersonalisation, loss of dignity, purpose and meaning, and the discouragement of meaningful social (and sexual) relationships. In addition, work by researchers such as Seligman (1975) and Brown and Harris (1978) led to a growing awareness of the psychological damage that social isolation and an enduring sense of loss of control could inflict upon the individual. Such well-founded concerns led to the development of the concept of *normalisation* (Wolfensberger 1972) and the belief that young adults with learning disabilities would benefit from living independently, either as individuals or in small group homes. This idea was extended beyond those living in institutions, to young people with learning disabilities living at home with their parents or adopted family (Reiter and Bendov 1996). This practice, it was argued, would integrate individuals with learning disabilities into society and reverse the social marginalisation that had occurred in the past (Smith 1995).

Rather ironically, one of the key normalisation concepts, *choice*, was not always offered to the individuals concerned (Reiter and Bendov 1996). Rather, it was taken for granted (with little supporting research) that community-living would proffer more advantages than disadvantages for individuals with learning disabilities. According to Smith (1995), many studies have shown that community care has failed to achieve key objectives, such as social integration at the level of the community and the facilitation of meaningful, close social relationships with others. Smith (1993), for example, found that many community-based participants rated staff, or rarely seen relatives, as their closest friends, whilst Firth and Rapley (1990) found that, despite the implementation of community-based programmes, few people in the community actually chose to spend time with the 'devalued'. Furthermore, Masters and Smith (1987) point out that, in line with *relative deprivation theory*, the negative effects of low socio-economic status may actually have been enhanced by an increased awareness of the contrast between those that have (quality of life) and those who do not.

Whilst these findings paint a rather bleak picture, they do need to be weighed against the many, and often profound, disadvantages that institutionalised care can entail. However, the primary lesson we should learn from this is to avoid the assumption that health professionals always know what is best for individuals.

Improving QOL

In considering QOL, we run up against a problem that we have encountered before: the individual's perception of reality does not always match that of the health professionals (Bowling 1991). For example, an environment can be objectively assessed as clean, safe and aesthetically pleasant, but it is the extent to which the individual is satisfied with it that is the critical factor (Schalock *et al.* 1990). This is the nub of the matter and it should impinge on all nursing decisions that have potentially major ramifications for individuals' lives. If an individual is happy in a relatively impoverished environment, who has the right to suggest that another would be better? Conversely, if an individual's environment impedes his or her personal dignity, autonomy, privacy and self-development, should health professionals not have a duty to improve that environment where possible?

Such issues are particularly salient when an expert has access to information or resources that could improve QOL for the individual whose ability to make an informed and rational choice is impaired due to cognitive impairment, illness, chronic institutionalisation or social anxiety. However, there are no easy solutions to such problems. As a nurse, your job should always be to act as the patient/client's advocate and to try and ensure that decisions are taken in the interest of improving the individual's QOL, regardless of whether the event involves a controversial treatment for cancer or a decision about whether to opt for community or institutionalised care.

Summary

Encouraging individuals to be vigilant about potential signs and symptoms of illness is an important element of primary or preventative health care. In general, the likelihood of symptom detection is increased when symptoms involve discomfort, pain and embarrassment, though others factors such as competing stimuli and the individual's emotional state also play an important mediating role. Even when symptoms are detected, however, the decision to seek professional help will depend upon the individual's perception or appraisal of the symptoms' meaning. This process of appraisal may be affected by cultural factors, individual factors, such as personal levels of knowledge, gender and age, and the extent to which the symptoms evoke fear and anxiety.

A number of theoretical models have been constructed to explain and predict the extent to which individuals will engage in health protective behaviours under a variety of circumstances. Of these, two of the most commonly referred-to models include the health belief model and the theory of reasoned action. According to the former model, factors such as perceived vulnerability and susceptibility and costs versus benefits play an important role in determining whether the individual will engage in health protective behaviours such as screening and immunisation. The latter model places emphasis on the role of others in determining in which behaviours the individual will eventually engage.

Finally, a general criticism of 'social cognition' models, such as the HBM and the TRA, is that they take little account of the role of factors such as stress and anxiety in decision-making processes. It is argued that these can lead to panic, denial and avoidance, which ultimately impair rational decision-making.

Chapter 11

Compliance and non-compliance with medical advice

Learning outcomes

By the end of this chapter you should be able to:

- Describe the basic causes of non-compliance.
- Describe how compliance may be achieved.
- Outline why the health professional should always take account of the patient's perspective.

Extent of the problem

Up until the 1970s, health practitioners had generally assumed that patients dutifully carried out their instructions, and little or no thought was given to the real extent of *compliance* with medical or health advice (Meichenbaum and Turk 1986). However, several pieces of research generated during this period shattered this illusion, by revealing that non-compliance was, in fact, commonplace.

It was found, for example, that compliance for treatment regimes involving behavioural change was as low as 15 per cent, whilst non-compliance with medication regimes was as high as 35 per cent (DiMatteo and DiNichola 1982; Steptoe and Mathews 1984; Meichenbaum and Turk 1986; Pitts 1991). In addition to these worrying statistics, Ley (1982) estimated that as many as one in five hospital admissions might result from non-compliance with health advice.

In the following discussion, we will seek to identify the principal causes of non-compliance and to examine how compliance can best be achieved. (Some authors prefer the term *adherence*, because it is less suggestive of a command and implies more of an interactional process between the health professional and patient.)

Understanding non-compliance

Two specific trends, or patterns, in non-compliance emerge from the literature. The first is that non-compliance increases in line with the *complexity of treatment regimes*. For example, Stone (1979) found that patient non-compliance rates for the administration of a regime involving one drug was typically around 15 per cent, rising to 25 per cent for two drugs and 35 per cent for three or more drugs. The second pattern to emerge from the literature is that compliance invariably *declines over time* and is particularly notable with chronic conditions, such as diabetes mellitus. Watts (1979), for example, found that non-compliance with Type 1, insulin dependent diabetes is typically around

50 per cent, and Meichenbaum and Turk (1986) report that the incidence of dosage error in insulin self-administration during the first five years is about 30 per cent, rising to 80 per cent for individuals who have had diabetes for twenty years or more.

In more general terms, however, non-compliance is highest when the condition is *chronic, but non-life threatening* and when the treatment is *prophylactic* and *requires changes in lifestyle and personal habits*. In addition, a number of specific factors, or classes of variable, have been shown significantly to influence compliance; these include attributional bias, health beliefs, treatment variables, the patient–practitioner relationship and organisational variables.

Attributional bias

Research has revealed that health professionals often blame the patient, rather than themselves, for patient non-compliance. For example, Davis (1968) found that medical practitioners typically attributed non-compliance to negative personality traits, such as the patient being weak-willed, lazy or unintelligent, and Stone (1979) found that only 25 per cent of general physicians believed that they might personally have a significant effect on compliance.

This tendency to blame the patient, rather than the self, may be a reflection of a deeper and more fundamental aspect of the way in which we process social information. For example, according to the *fundamental attribution bias*, we typically attribute other people's behaviour to internal, *person variables*, rather than to external, *situational variables* (Ross *et al.* 1977). For instance, a nurse may unthinkingly attribute a doctor's brusque instructions to arrogance and conceit, rather than to the effects of working a 72 hour shift.

Although such attributional biases are generally viewed as automatic and pre-conscious, it is clear that, by blaming the other person, the health professional absolves him or her self from personal responsibility and is also freed from a potentially time-consuming exploration of the situational factors that may have contributed to the patient's behaviour. In fact, researchers have found little evidence to support the notion of a 'non-compliant personality' (Seltzer and Hoffman 1980) and it appears that other factors, such as the individual's prior knowledge of illness, have a far greater effect on compliance than either personality or levels of intelligence (DiMatteo and DiNichola 1982; Meichenbaum and Turk 1986).

Health beliefs

Patients often hold theories or *beliefs* about the causes and consequences of illness, which can vary in their levels of accuracy (Zola 1981). Sometimes these beliefs are based upon a poor understanding of the body's systems and sometimes they are based upon cultural myths. Furthermore, even when the practitioner and patient appear to share the same terminology, there is a risk that the different lay and medical meanings attached to terms will result in both parties talking (in blissful ignorance) about quite different things! For this reason alone, it is particularly important that the patient's health beliefs are fully explored.

When dealing with patients, it is wise to adopt the position that they typically enter treatment with some *knowledge* of the nature of their problem, together with *expectations* about treatment and outcomes. In order to explore these beliefs, it is essential that patients are afforded the opportunity to express what they believe to be the cause(s) of their symptoms, how they feel these should be treated, and what effects they think treatment may have on their lives and on those around them. By exploring these beliefs, you are afforded the opportunity to challenge any misperceptions that may otherwise affect compliance with heath advice post-consultation.

Meichenbaum and Turk (1986, p. 47) provide good examples of the type of beliefs that can undermine compliance:

- You need to give your body a rest from medicine once in a while or otherwise your body becomes too dependent upon it or immune to it.
- I resent being controlled by drugs.
- God will take care of my illness.
- I do too many preventative things to be susceptible to illness.
- My depression is biological, there is nothing I can do.
- How will I know if I still need them if I keep taking the pills?

When exploring health beliefs, it is important to remember that patients and carers often have useful ideas that may aid their recovery. This is particularly likely when dealing with individuals who have in-depth knowledge relating to some long-standing condition. It is also important that the effects that the treatment may have on the individual, and on those close to or dependent upon them, are fully explored. In fact, we can relate this point back to the HBM, by stating that the patient is unlikely to comply with a treatment regime if he or she perceives that the costs are likely to outweigh the benefits (Janz and Becker 1984).

In general, research has shown that perceived vulnerability is positively correlated with compliance (Becker and Rosenstock 1984). However, as noted earlier, anxiety about possible outcomes may lead to denial or avoidance of the condition and subsequent non-compliance when the patient feels vulnerable and threatened (Antonovosky and Hartman 1974). Such non-compliance may be regarded as logical and rational viewed from the patient's perspective, because it relieves them from anxiety. However, the corresponding actions may be viewed as illogical and irrational by the health practitioner, who may regard denial as a dubious short-term 'head in the sand' solution. These conflicting points of view demonstrate the need to consider the patient's perspective when proposing treatment.

Rotter's *locus of control theory* (1966) has been used by health researchers to investigate the hypothesis that individuals' beliefs about their ability to control events significantly affect compliance. According to the original theory, individuals high in an *internal locus of control* (LOC) believe that they have the ability to control events around them, whilst individuals high in an *external locus of control* believe that they have little personal influence over life events. Applying this rationale, researchers attempted to show that those high in an internal LOC would be more likely to comply with medical advice, because they believed that their actions would result directly in benefits to health, whilst those high in an external LOC would be less likely to comply with health advice, because they were fatalistic. Although subsequent research did find support for this hypothesis, in that individuals high in an internal LOC tended to be more active in their own treatment, evidence also emerged that they were just as likely to modify treatment regimes, *because* they wanted to feel in control. De Vellis *et al.* (1980), for example, found that high internal LOC individuals being treated for epilepsy were more likely to reduce, or stop, their anti-convulsant medication in order to explore what the outcome would be.

The latter represents a case of *rational non-compliance*, which typically occurs when the patient wishes to regain a sense of control or mastery or when the disadvantages posed by side effects are deemed to outweigh the advantages of treatment. Rosenhan and Seligman (1995), for example, note that individuals suffering from other mental health disorders, such as schizophrenia, sometimes stop taking medication to see if the active symptoms have subsided or gone away, and similarly Kaplan *et al.* (1993) report that male patients showed a reluctance to continue the use of hypotensive drugs because of side effects such as sexual impotence.

Recognising this need for control is important, and treatment regimes should always be tailored towards helping individuals to attain this goal (perhaps with the exception of acutely ill patients who have a short-term need to relinquish control to powerful others).

Treatment variables

We learnt earlier that non-compliance is frequently associated with complex treatment regimes, which are sometimes necessitated by chronic conditions. It has been suggested that such regimes can lead to a state of *information overload*, which may result in a failure to grasp instructions and cause the patient to subsequently modify, delay or simply avoid implementing the requirements of the regime (Ley and Spelman 1967; DiMatteo and DiNichola 1982). In order to minimise the likelihood of this occurring, it is important that you are able to provide patients with information that is specifically tailored to their needs and abilities, and it may be desirable to provide the information in stages, if the patient is excessively anxious, distracted and unreceptive.

Individuals are particularly reluctant to engage in regimes that require the cessation of habitual behaviours that are pleasurable or positively reinforcing (Steptoe and Mathews 1984). Patients may, for example, be unwilling to give up smoking if they believe that it helps to 'steady their nerves' or keeps their weight down. In such cases, you should first identify any 'target behaviours' that the patient may find difficult to relinquish and then negotiate a partial, or gradual, reduction in them, if a total cessation is deemed unlikely. In consideration of this point, it is worth remembering that it is easier to replace some pleasurable activity, like smoking or drinking, if the patient can find some positively reinforcing alternative.

Under certain conditions, illness can result in over-compliance and adherence to the *sick role* (Parsons 1951). This is particularly likely to occur when individuals have experienced some chronic condition that results in them being highly dependent upon others for their basic needs over a period of months or years. For example, an individual hospitalised with chronic pain, or depression, may slip into a submissive role that involves a diminution of personal responsibility and the acceptance of a more passive role.

Patients are often reluctantly forced into the sick role, because of untoward events; however, after a time they learn that it can afford them *secondary gains* that are intrinsically reinforcing (Fordyce 1976). The *institutionalised* mental health or learning disabilities patient, for example, may benefit through not having to think about cooking or cleaning, or having to work or take responsibility for themselves or others. This role may appear particularly attractive to people who, for whatever reason, have come to doubt their ability to function adequately in their day to day lives. Non-compliance may present a means of being able to ensure that such benefits are not removed. This is a particularly difficult problem to overcome and it is sometimes managed by instituting a behavioural treatment programme (such as may be employed in chronic pain clinics) that positively reinforces 'well behaviours' (such as taking responsibility for identified tasks) with praise and encouragement. (Note that institutionalisation and learned helplessness are similar but unique psychological constructs. The institutionalised patient's passive and compliant behaviour is positively reinforced by the staff and by the rules and structure of the institution. Learned helplessness, however, is a condition that is caused by a personal, perceived loss of control that is not necessarily reinforced by members of staff.)

Patient–practitioner relationship

Practitioners from all health disciplines have an important role to play in helping the individual to achieve and maintain optimal compliance. This can be facilitated by providing patients with clear, honest explanations and advice and by being sensitive to their individual needs (Pitts 1991). It is also important to avoid technical jargon that may be meaningless to the patient. For example, I recall that a conversation with a group of patients in an acute psychiatric ward revealed that they were baffled and somewhat bemused by the term *primary nurse*. On admission, they had all been allocated to one, but nobody had thought it necessary to explain what the role of the primary nurse was. Although they laughed about this in retrospect, one patient admitted that she had suffered in silence for a whole weekend, because she had mistakenly believed that she was allowed to talk only to her primary nurse.

In a similar vein, we should avoid using ambiguous instructions and jargon. The following examples adapted from Zola (1981, pp. 247–248) show how confusion can arise when the patient tries to carry out their general practitioner's instructions at home:

*GP: *Take the drug four times a day.*
Patient: Does this mean I should take it every six hours? Do I need to wake up in the middle of the night and what if I forget to take a dose, should I double the next dosage?

*GP: *Keep your leg elevated most of the day.*
Patient: How high is elevated? How long is most of the day? What should I do when I'm asleep?

*GP: *Come back if there are any complications.*
Patient: What is a complication and how will I know what symptoms are related to the disease and what to the treatment?

Although the latter examples are inserted to provide a little light relief, they should alert you to the need to avoid similarly meaningless rhetoric when practising as a health professional.

Communication and compliance

There is evidence that non-compliance is often caused by poor communication, and the issues involved have been highlighted succinctly by DiMatteo and DiNichola (1982) who found that:

- Patients typically forget the bulk of information supplied to them.
- The diagnosis is often retained, whilst instructions and advice are forgotten.
- The more information that is given, the more is forgotten.
- Information provided at the start and finish of consultation is more likely to be remembered than that included in the middle. (The so-called *primacy-recency effect*).
- Individual differences in intelligence have little effect on recall of instructions, whilst prior knowledge of illness does.
- High states of arousal (as caused by anxiety) have an adverse effect on recall.

It follows, therefore, that you should always seek to give information and advice in a clear and concise manner and ensure that important instructions are given at the start of a consultation and repeated towards the end. Additionally, the patient's emotional state should be considered and efforts should be made to avoid overloading the patient with information when he or she is in a state of high anxiety.

Organisational variables

Geersten *et al.* (1973) found that patient compliance decreased as waiting times for consultation increased. For example, 67 per cent of patients waiting between thirty minutes and one hour were subsequently found to be compliant, whilst the figure dropped to only 31 per cent for those waiting in excess of one hour. Similarly, there is evidence that the use of individualised appointment times in outpatient clinics results in better compliance than block-booking appointment systems (Pitts 1991).

The improvements in compliance found with more personalised systems is probably due to an increase in trust and confidence in the practitioner and enhanced feelings of self-worth. Applying this rationale, it seems likely that individualised care systems, such as those employing a primary or key nurse, will result in greater levels of compliance than that obtained through systems relying heavily on task-orientated care. In addition, the increased nurse–patient contact is likely to facilitate a greater awareness of the patient's perspective and beliefs about treatment outcomes, which may help to promote compliance.

Finally, there is evidence that increased supervision of patients nursed at home can also lead to increased compliance, particularly when the condition is chronic. Garrity and Garrity (1985) speculate that this may be due to increased social support and personal concern about the patient's condition, a greater awareness of the patient's problems and enhancement of the patient's problem-solving skills.

Summary

The decision to seek professional help for physical and psychological problems is dependent upon the individual being aware that something is amiss. This is most likely to happen when symptoms are unusual, painful or cause distress and discomfort. When symptoms are detected, it is common to approach a colleague or friend to ask for their advice, and it is often prompts via this 'lay-referral system' that lead the patient to seek professional help.

Individuals may avoid seeking help from lay or professional sources when their condition carries a social stigma and/or is perceived to be embarrassing or shameful. Similarly, individuals may avoid seeking help when doing so evokes anxiety and the belief that treatment will involve costs that outweigh the potential benefits.

The HBM and the TRA are often employed to predict health protective behaviours, such as help-seeking behaviour for signs and symptoms of illness and participation in screening and vaccination programmes. According to the HBM, individuals are most likely to engage in health protective behaviour when they feel personally vulnerable and believe that the benefits of taking action outweigh the costs. The TRA suggests that stated intentions are better predictors of behaviour than attitudes or beliefs, and focuses on the importance of others' opinions and attitudes in respect of health behaviours.

Both the HBM and the TRA assume that decision-making is always logical and rational. However, there is evidence that decision-making under conditions of stress may become irrational and maladaptive when the individual lacks appropriate information about alternative courses of action or holds the belief that they lack time to enact a safe alternative. It follows, therefore, that in circumstances such as acute health crises, the models may have limited value in predicting the individual's behaviour.

Non-compliance with health advice is regarded as a potentially serious problem, which adversely affects the health of individuals and places unnecessary pressure on health resources. Non-compliance is most likely to occur when treatment regimes are prophylactic, complex and protracted, and when the patient's condition is non-life-threatening but chronic and difficult to treat successfully.

Health practitioners sometimes blame the patient for non-compliance. However, the evidence suggests that non-compliance is due to a broad range of factors, of which personality is only one. The tendency to attribute blame to the patient may be due to the fundamental attribution bias, which is an unconscious bias in information-processing that leads the observer to attribute blame to internal, person variables rather than to external, situational variables.

Patients generally enter or exit treatment with beliefs about the possible causes of symptoms and/or the outcomes of certain illness-related conditions. These health beliefs should always be fully explored in order to identify misconceptions and to maximise future compliance with health advice. However, directly challenging such beliefs can be counterproductive when the individual is unwilling, or unable, to relinquish them. Under such circumstances, compromise is often the best course of action.

Compliance is likely to be facilitated if the patient's treatment regime allows him or her to maintain a sense of personal control. However, non-compliance may sometimes be viewed as rational, given that it allows the patient a means of achieving perceived control. It should not, therefore, necessarily be frowned upon.

Communication is similarly important, and technical and ambiguous jargon should always be avoided and replaced with clear, concise instructions. You should seek to avoid information overload and be aware of the patient's emotional state when attempting to impart important advice or instructions. Information provided at the beginning and end of a consultation is more likely to be retained than that given in the middle.

You should be aware of the phenomenon labelled the 'sick role', and should avoid unintentionally reinforcing it by making the patient overly dependent upon you and other members of staff. 'Well behaviours' can be positively reinforced using simple praise and encouragement.

User-friendly systems appear to encourage compliance as they help to build up confidence and trust in the health professional. Such relationships should form the basis of all successful interventions.

MINI SELF-TEST

1   Describe the four factors that affect symptom detection.

2   Outline the importance of the lay-referral system in help-seeking behaviour.

3   Describe the six factors that are likely to affect the individual's perception of illness.

4   Outline the main factors contained in the Health Belief Model.

5   Explain why a knowledge of the patient's attitudes alone is often insufficient to allow accurate predictions of behaviour.

6   Describe the three factors that determine rational decision-making under conditions of stress.

7   Briefly list the factors that lead to non-compliance.

8   Briefly list the factors that facilitate optimal compliance.

REFLECTIVE SCENARIOS

Megan

Megan is a 39-year-old successful barrister who is married with two children. She is expecting her third child and is thirty-two weeks pregnant. During the past couple of weeks she has put on quite a lot of extra weight, has been experiencing headaches, swollen ankles and hands and she feels constantly tired.

Discuss the extent to which she may attribute these symptoms to her age and job or to possible symptoms of some underlying physical disorder with reference to symptom detection and perception.

Jorgen

Jorgen is a 25-year-old man who has learning disabilities. He has been living in sheltered accommodation for the past five years, where basic domestic services are provided by staff. He says he is happy there, but his day consists of little more than watching TV and smoking heavily. As a consequence, he has become quite obese and is lethargic and non-cooperative. His key worker thinks that he would benefit from a more challenging environment and there is a place available soon in a small house where residents share responsibilities for cooking, shopping and cleaning. His key worker believes he is capable of this, but Jorgen flatly refuses to consider moving.

Discuss this situation with reference to basic issues in QOL assessment.

Naomi

Naomi is 19 years old and has smoked around twenty to thirty cigarettes a day since the age of 14. Following a visit to her general practitioner for bronchitis, she is told that her life will be shortened by ten to fifteen years if she does not quit soon.

Discuss the factors that may influence whether or not she decides to quit or reduce the amount she smokes with reference to the Health Belief Model and the Theory of Reasoned Action.

Mary

Mary is a 45-year-old female with breast cancer. Her consultant has advised her to have a radical mastectomy, followed by a course of radio-therapy. As an afterthought, however, he adds that she could opt for a less disfiguring 'lumpectomy', but with a reduced chance of long-term survival.

With reference to 'making health decisions under conditions of stress', discuss what conditions will be necessary if she is to make an informed, rational choice.

Steven

Steven suffers from chronic schizophrenia, which is controlled by the use of depot injections (slow release major tranquillisers administered by regular injection). He has been completely well for eighteen months now and wants to stop the medication. His key worker advises him that it is the medication that keeps him symptom free, but Steven refuses to have his injection nonetheless.

Discuss the extent to which his actions represent rational non-compliance or a lack of insight.

Suggested reading

Banyard, P. (1996). *Applying Psychology to Health*. Coventry: Banyard Stoughton.
This is a health psychology text for health professionals that contains many informative chapters linking behaviour and health.

Bennet, P. and Murphy, S. (1997). *Psychology and Health Promotion*. Buckingham: Open University Press.
This is an informative text that provides an overview of the psychological factors that influence health behaviours.

Meichenbaum, D. and Turk, D. C. (1986). *Facilitating Treatment Adherence*. New York: Plenum Press.
This lucid text provides an excellent account of the factors that impede and facilitate compliance.

Stockwell, F. (1984). *The Unpopular Patient*. Beckenham: Crook-Helm Ltd.
The subject of nurse–patient relationships is largely beyond the scope of my text, though it is important in terms of compliance. Stockwell's text, although a little dated, highlights basic issues and is still worth reading.

Part four

Psycho-physiology: The relationship between mind and body

Chapter 12

Psycho-physiological reactions to acute and chronic stress

Learning outcomes

By the end of this chapter you should be able to:

- Outline the general adaptation syndrome.
- Describe how stress may affect the body's immune response.

There is now a considerable body of evidence showing that psychological factors can exert a direct effect on the body's physiological systems. In this section, we will focus on three specific topics that are of direct relevance to nursing practice. The first examines the effects that stress can have on the body and the immune system. The second explores the role that personality type may play in the aetiology of major diseases, such as coronary heart disease and cancer, and the third focuses on the role that psychological factors play in mediating the experience of pain, with special reference to models of pain.

The general adaptation syndrome

Seyle (1979) was one of the first investigators to identify a common pattern of physiological response to acute and chronic stress, which he termed the *general adaptation syndrome*, or GAS for short. According to the model, exposure to stress activates the sympathetic nervous system (SNS), which results in subsequent progression through three stages of physiological response:

Stage 1. Alarm reaction

During the initial *alarm stage*, the release of the neurotransmitters *epinephrine* and *norepinephrine* results in an increase in blood pressure and heart rate as the body is prepared for extraordinary levels of activity. Such high levels of arousal cannot be maintained, however, and if the stressor is still present, the stress response moves into the second stage.

Stage 2. Resistance

During this second stage, *resistance*, the high levels of arousal that characterised the initial response are reduced to lower levels that, nonetheless, still lie above the norm, and *corticosteroids*, or 'stress hormones', are released as the body attempts to resist or combat the stressor. Whilst the individual may no longer be aware that they are stressed, the body's reserve stores of fat and carbohydrates are slowly being depleted, and damage caused to the body's systems results in the emergence of *diseases of adaptation*, such as hypertension, eczema and diabetes.

Stage 3. Exhaustion

During the final stage, *exhaustion*, the body's reserves are finally spent and the damage to the cardiovascular or immune system results in some condition, such as stroke, myocardial infarction, cancer or bacterial infection.

GAS and emotional specificity

Although Seyle believed that the GAS reaction was non-specific (i.e. that it would be elicited equally by physical and psychological stressors), there is evidence that epinephrine, norepinephrine and corticosteroids are most likely to be released when a strong *emotional reaction* is evoked (Sarrafino 1994). Such reactions are likely to be evoked by stressful events, such as bereavement, which may partially explain the typical increase in morbidity and mortality found during the first six to twelve months post-bereavement (Carr 1982). By the same token, acute physical and psychological health crises are also likely to evoke strong emotional reactions in individuals, which may well impede recovery if the sequelae result in chronic stress.

An evolutionary perspective

Exactly why the body's response to stress should have the potential to reap such negative consequences has been the subject of some debate, leading to the suggestion that the stress response is *maladaptive* viewed from the perspective of modern man (Rosenhan and Seligman 1995). To understand why this may be, we need to adopt an evolutionary perspective. Imagine, for example, that as caveman, or cavewoman, you come to face to face with some prehistoric nasty. Your heart pounds as the alarm response is triggered, and with heroic exertion you find the resources to fight or flee your foe. Shortly afterwards, homeostasis returns, you put some more sticks on the fire and settle down for a restful night's sleep. However, now imagine yourself as a 1990s stressed-out office worker facing probable redundancy or as a hospitalised patient awaiting surgery for advanced cancer. You cannot easily fight or flee your foe, because the enemy is an internal feeling of personal inadequacy or the fear of an invisible physiological process that you can'not directly see or control. Furthermore, unlike the primitive animals in which the stress response has its evolutionary roots, you are not locked in the here and now. You have the ability to fantasise and reflect on what may happen, and when these premonitions are negative, you are filled with anticipatory anxiety that feeds an ongoing cycle of stress.

Whilst this may sound a touch melodramatic, it should serve to illustrate why the body's stress response can work against us. Of course, people do learn to cope with adverse events by minimising the perceived risk or threats to the self through the use of mental defence mechanisms or illusory self-perceptions. Yet such mechanisms are not always successful and, as we will now learn, there is a considerable body of evidence that points to a strong link between chronic stress and ill health.

Stress and immunocompetence

The immune system

The immune system has two primary functions: it has to recognise foreign substances, or *antigens*, present on surface membranes and structures of things like viruses and bacteria, and it must disable them and remove them from the body. The system can be split into two parts: a non-specific and a specific response. The *non-specific immune response* prevents the entry of antigens via the skin or mucous membranes and prevents the spread of infection. The *specific immune response* targets specific antigens that have gained access to the body in the following way:

A group of specific defence cells termed *B cells*, *T cells* and *NK (natural killer) cells*, circulate in the blood stream of healthy individuals and destroy antigens by the following means:

1   When a foreign antigen is encountered for the first time, B cells produce antibodies that are specific to it. These antibodies disable the antigen by locking on to structures on its surface.

2   T cells also target specific antigens and destroy them by multi-
     plying in number and lysing (breaking down) the foreign cell
     membrane. They may also remove the antigen, engulfing it by
     phagocytosis.
3   The immune system retains memory cells for previously encoun-
     tered antigens and can quickly reproduce a specific response to
     destroy them.
4   NK cells also remove foreign antibodies, but are thought to be
     particularly important in detecting and destroying tumours.

Assessing immunocompetence

The body's *immunocompetence*, or its ability to deal with antigens, can
be easily assessed in a variety of ways, which include counting the number and type of T cells present in the blood (sometimes referred to as
white blood cells), or assessing skin reactions to the deliberate injection
of antigens (the greater the reaction, the better the immune response).
When the body's immune response is compromised, there may be
insufficient numbers of immune cells in the blood stream to deal with
invaders, or the body may be unable to reproduce specific antibodies
rapidly to deal with previously encountered pathogens.

Evidence supporting a link between stress and impaired immunocompetence

Kiecolt-Glaser *et al.* (1984) found that medical students had lowered
NK cell activity on the day of their finals compared to a matched
control group. In addition, they found a positive correlation between
the reported stressfulness of the event and lowered NK activity. Irwin
et al. (1987) found that bereavement was associated with a reduction in
NK activity and a lower T cell count. Similarly, Bartrop *et al.* (1977)
found a lowered T cell count in bereaved spouses at a six-week follow
up post-bereavement. McKinnon *et al.* (1989) found lower levels of
B, NK and T cell activity in Three Mile Island residents, following the
much publicised radiation leak in their locality, as compared to a
matched control group. Fawzy *et al.* (1993) found that cancer sufferers
who were offered psychological interventions, such as problem-solving
and relaxation techniques, had lower rates of mortality at six month and

six year follow ups, compared to controls who were not offered the interventions.

Kiecolt-Glaser and Glaser (1995) state that exactly how stress mechanisms result in an impaired immune system is not fully understood, though it is suggested that the release of stress hormones suppresses the efficiency of the thymus gland, which directs immune activity. There is, however, also evidence that a loss of emotional support can suppress the immune system by means not yet fully understood. For example, Berkman (1995) reports that individuals caring for a partner with Alzheimer's disease showed evidence of continued impaired immunocompetence even when their partners were placed into temporary residential care, suggesting that it is the loss of emotional support inherent in caring for a partner with dementia that causes the damage and not the stress of caring *per se*. If her assumptions are correct, health professionals have a further pressing reason for examining how vulnerable individuals, such as carers, may be adequately supported when they lack the emotional support that their partner was once able to offer.

Third factor variables

Although the evidence seems impressive, it should be treated with a measure of caution, because the effects could be due to the presence of *third factor variables* that were not controlled for in the latter studies. For example, although bereavement is associated with impaired immunocompetence, it is also associated with an increase in alcohol consumption (Rosenhan and Seligman 1995), and it is known that heavy to moderate alcohol consumption can lower T cell toxicity or the cell's destructive effectiveness (Gatchel *et al.* 1989). Similarly, inattention to diet, inactivity, or increased smoking are all behavioural responses that are associated with stressful life events and impairment of the body's immune response (Kiecolt-Glaser and Glaser 1995).

In fact, Kiecolt-Glaser and Glaser (1995) suggest that we can predict that stress will affect immunocompetence with surety only when the individual's immune system is *already* compromised, as may occur, for example, in individuals with Acquired Immune Deficiency Syndrome (AIDS) or in the elderly. In support of this hypothesis, they point out that immunocompetence declines as a function of age, and that the elderly are particularly likely to die of opportunist infectious diseases, such as pneumonia and influenza. Similarly, they point out that older adults are more likely to show impaired immune functions in association with depression than younger adults.

A model of impaired immune functioning

Taking what we have learnt so far, we can build a simple model that demonstrates how stressful life events may conceivably lead to the development of disease (see Table 12.1). According to the model, a major life event, such as bereavement, threatens the individual's psychological and physical well-being. This leads to feelings of vulnerability and perceived helplessness, which may eventually result in depression. These emotional responses, or states, trigger the release of stress hormones that compromise the body's immune response, with the result that the body is subsequently unable to mount an effective response to exposure to pathogens or mutating cells. The net result of this chain of events is the development of disease.

TABLE 12.1 A model of stress-impaired immunocompetence and disease

Stage	Characteristics
1	Stressful event
2	Perceived helplessness
3	Depression
4	Release of stress hormones
5	Impaired immunocompetence
6	Exposure to a pathogen or mutating cell goes unchecked
7	Resulting disease.

Focus on clinical practice: stress and self-awareness

Causes of stress

Stress has been described as endemic in western societies, and a wide range of causes have been identified that include challenging life events, self-doubt and negative self-appraisal, overwork, excessive emotional demands, time pressure, exams, parenthood, disturbed sleep, new work environment, difficulty in balancing roles, and relationship problems, to name but a few. No doubt many of you reading this text will recognise at least some of these pressures in your own lives. However, as we have already learnt, it is often not events themselves that cause stress and anxiety, but rather the way in which we perceive them and deal with them (Lazarus and Folkman 1984). Unfortunately, stress can be insidious, building gradually, so that individuals are unaware that they are suffering from it. Consequently, the first step in effective personal stress management is to recognise the basic signs and symptoms that can inform us when we are subjected (or are subjecting ourselves) to excessive physical and emotional stress.

Detecting signs of stress

The *physiological stress response* is broadly composed of a *short-term response*, mediated by the action of the sympathetic nervous system (i.e. the release of epinephrine and norepinephrine), and a *long-term response*, mediated by the endocrine system (i.e. the release of corticosteroids). The short-term physical response may be recognised by symptoms such as an increase in heart rate, insomnia, chest pain, nausea, diarrhoea and stomach ache, and the long-term physical responses by a diverse range of symptoms that include feeling generally rundown, weight gain or loss, susceptibility to bacterial and viral infections, loss of libido, muscle pain, menstrual irregularity, bowel irritability, reduction in mobility and heart disease (Davidson and Neale 1982; Bennet and Murphy 1997).

The *psychological stress response* broadly encompasses our *emotions, cognitions* and *behaviour,* and may be recognised by the presence of symptoms such as impatience and increased irritability, frequent feelings of anger and aggressive outbursts, being easily upset by minor changes, rumination, being unable to 'switch off', excessive use of drugs (such as alcohol) to wind down, poor decision-making, blaming others,

PSYCHO-PHYSIOLOGICAL REACTIONS

cynicism, job dissatisfaction, avoidance behaviour and low feelings of self-worth (Marks 1987).

Checking thoughts, actions and feelings

Simmons and Daw (1994) suggest that effective stress management is underpinned by self-awareness of the types of event that trigger stress and of our thoughts, feelings and subsequent actions.

Triggers

Once you have become adept at detecting physical and psychological cues that indicate the existence of stress, the first step is to learn what type of events function as triggers or antecedents. This may be achieved by making mental (or written) notes about the type of events that result in stress during the course of a normal day and comparing them over a period of time.

Thoughts

The next step involves making a note of the thoughts that occur during such events. Do you, for example, talk yourself down with thoughts such as, 'I know I am going to make a mess of this', or do you ruminate incessantly after the event, repeatedly telling yourself how foolish you were for not having handled the event more adeptly, or do you shift responsibility to a third party, in effect blaming others for the way you feel?

Feelings

It is also helpful to make a note of your feelings during the event. Do you, for example, react to the situation with feelings of anxiety, irritation, anger, sadness or a sense of hopelessness?

Actions

Finally, make a note of how you react to the situation. Do you, for example, get verbally or physically aggressive or do you avoid the situation by making excuses and hiding out of the way? Do you drink, eat or smoke more in response to the event? Do you try to ignore the event by pretending it is not happening or by diverting your attention elsewhere?

Coping positively with stressors

Irrational responses

As I am sure you are well aware, stressors are part and parcel of everyday life and it is impossible to avoid stress completely. However, the negative effects of stressors may be greatly increased when underpinned by irrational beliefs or faulty thinking (Ellis 1962; Beck and Emery 1985). In such cases, professional help may be sought to help the individual identify negative thoughts and to replace them with more positive ones. This is largely done through self-instruction and self-statement training (Meichenbaum 1977), though in some cases longer-term psycho-therapy or assertiveness training may be indicated if the root-cause of the problem is a chronically low self-esteem.

This aside, all of us engage in faulty thinking from time to time. A student may, for example, feel a complete failure on the basis of a single assessment failure, whilst one poor placement report (particularly when it comes early in the course) may lead the student to conclude that he or she will never make a good nurse.

The trick is to recognise negative self-statements or thoughts, put things in context and think of the positive aspects of self that we all possess.

Rational responses

Sometimes feelings such as anxiety and a sense of powerlessness may be viewed as wholly rational responses to stressful and seemingly uncontrollable situations. However, it is often possible to adopt a problem-solving approach to dealing with such stressors. Such techniques involve *redefining the stressor* and breaking the problem down into its constituent parts (Simmons and Daw 1994). These can then be prioritised and dealt with as a series of short- and long-term objectives or goals. For example, extreme emotional stress, or *burnout*, of staff working in an emotionally demanding environment, such as palliative care, may be dealt with by first identifying the primary stressors and then developing short-term procedures to deal with them. At a team level, this might include encouraging the use of stress recognition and management techniques and by working towards longer-term objectives, such as regular individual supervision and appraisal, staff rotation, examining nursing procedures and team relationships, etc.

Stress and the patient

Techniques for dealing with stress, such as problem-solving and self-statement training, are useful for patients too, particularly when they are suffering from depression in response to some event that results in low self-esteem. Splitting one large problem into smaller parts usually makes it easier to deal with, and short-term, attainable goals can be set, which help to boost self-confidence. However, the bottom line is that, when dealing with patients, it is important that you are alert to the signs and symptoms of stress in yourself. If you cannot care for yourself properly, the quality of your work and your relationship with patients and other members of staff is very likely to suffer.

Personality type and disease

Personality and disease

The belief that physique, personality and disease are interlinked has an impressive history dating back to the Ancient Greeks, who believed, for example, that the melancholic, or depressive, personality was associated with an excess of black bile. In a similar vein, the works of Shakespeare also reflected the belief that body type was linked to personality. For example, Caesar is heard to comment on Cassius, 'Yond Cassius has a lean and hungry look; he thinks too much: such men are dangerous' (*Julius Caesar* act 1, scene 2). More recently, Sheldon (1954) equated the slightly plump, or endomorphic, body shape with a relaxed and sociable temperament, and Alexander (1950) proposed that specific types of *psychodynamic conflict* could result in certain types of disease in individuals who were genetically predisposed, arguing, for example, that genetically vulnerable individuals would develop peptic ulcers if they frequently experienced conflict between autonomy and dependency needs.

Whilst research has failed to offer convincing evidence in support of the latter 'theories', Grace and Graham's (1952) proposal that *specific thought patterns* might precipitate certain types of illness is reflected in much of the recent thinking on the relationship between mind and body. They suggested, for example, that being in a constant state of preparedness to deal with threats could lead to chronic hypertension. This line of thought bears much resemblance to current hypotheses about the relationship between stress and heart disease, as we will discover next.

Type A personality or behaviour and coronary heart disease

The current surge of interest in the relationship between personality and disease can be traced back to research carried out by two cardiologists, Friedman and Rosenman, during the 1960s and 1970s. They were interested in the idea that certain personality traits might cause, or increase, the risk of coronary heart disease (CHD), and they went on to develop a theory that proposed that individuals displaying *Type A behaviour* were more likely to develop CHD than those displaying *Type B behaviour.*

According to the theory, Type A behaviour is composed of the following three components of behavioural response that are habitually expressed across a wide range of situations. Given this, the Type A construct is much more akin to a personality trait than a simple pattern of behaviour, though it is less frequently referred to as a trait.

Competitiveness and achievement-oriented behaviour

Type As are strongly motivated to reach goals that are difficult to attain. They are highly competitive and are rarely satisfied with their achievements.

Time urgency and impatience

Type As feel under constant pressure to get things done and are typically driven by the belief that there is insufficient time to achieve their aims. They tend to talk and act quickly and their impatience can lead to errors, which causes them further pressure.

Hostility and aggressiveness

Although not physically aggressive, Type As are inclined to be impatient and irritable and to display a hostile attitude towards others who block their goals. Their social interactions often create conflict, which can result in correspondingly competitive or aggressive behaviour in those around them. In addition, Type As are concerned about losing control (Glass 1977) and this fear drives them to try and achieve more in order to attain a sense of relief.

Type B behaviour

As you may have already guessed, Type B people display the opposite personality traits (i.e. they tend to be less competitive, less aggressive, more patient, etc.) and have a much lower risk of heart disease than Type As. Echoing a comment made earlier in this text, however, it is worth noting that investigators have been relatively uninterested in exploring whether specific characteristics of the Type B personality might actually help prevent heart disease.

Evidence supporting the link between Type A behaviour and coronary heart disease

The hypothesis that Type A behaviour is a significant risk factor for coronary heart disease (CHD) has been contested, because several large and well-conducted studies have resulted in conflicting evidence. Friedman and Rosenman (1960), for example, conducted an eight-year *longitudinal study* of 3,400 healthy, middle-class males, and determined that Type As were twice as likely to develop CHD as Type Bs; a further large study carried out by Haynes *et al.* (1980) found a similar risk for middle-class males and females. However, other large studies (e.g. Cohen and Reed 1984 and Mathews and Haynes 1986) failed to show that Type A behaviour was a significant risk factor for CHD, and a twenty-two-year follow up of the males employed in Friedman and Rosenman's original study found that an increased risk of CHD was associated with smoking, raised systolic blood pressure and serum cholesterol, but *not* with Type A behaviour.

Despite these problems, most researchers in the field agree that there is such a considerable body of evidence supporting the Type A–CHD link that *something* is causing the excess risk found in so many large and well-conducted studies. For this reason, researchers have recently turned their attentions towards the individual components of the Type A construct, and the component that has been singled out is *hostility and aggression*, or HO for short. Literature reviews carried out by Smith (1992) and Whiteman *et al.* (1997) have found evidence of a consistent link between HO and increased risk of CHD, and this link is further supported by the finding that habitually hostile individuals react more intensely to social stressors, perceive them more frequently as threats and create stressful situations by their very behaviour (Williams and Barefoot 1988). In short, the stress generated by the HO individual's perceptions and responses is likely to fuel the chronic hypertension and long-term wear and tear on coronary arteries that precipitate CHD.

Despite this evidence, not all authorities are convinced that HO is an important causal variable. Conduit (1992), for instance, suggests that

PSYCHO-PHYSIOLOGY

situational variables, such as bereavement, are much more powerful predictors of CHD than personality variables, and argues that clinicians should concentrate on these instead. However, like many issues in psychology, the real debate is much more complex. Scheier and Bridges (1995), for example, point out that personality traits may only be expressed in certain (i.e. stressful) situations. So HO might be evident only in the aftermath of some major, debilitating condition, such as CHD.

Given the circular nature of this problem, it is best to view CHD (and other major diseases for that matter) as *multi-factorial*, or caused by an interaction of multiple factors, which would include not only personality and coping style, but also gender, age, lifestyle and genetic vulnerability.

Other personality variables linked to disease

Pessimism and fatalism

The terms *pessimism* and *fatalism* refer to the habitual tendency to expect the worst possible outcome when things go wrong. Research has shown that this personality characteristic is associated with an increase in *morbidity* and *mortality* in patients suffering from serious illness. Reed *et al.* (1994), for example, found that survival time in male patients with AIDS was negatively correlated with fatalism, and that having a positive attitude increased life expectancy. Similarly, Shultz *et al.* (1994) examined cancer patients receiving palliative radiation treatment and found a positive correlation between pessimism and death in younger patients aged 30–39. In addition, Scheier and Carver (1985) found evidence that pessimism was significantly correlated with perioperative myocardial infarction.

Emotional suppression or Type C behaviour

Emotional suppression refers to the habitual tendency to suppress one's emotions rather than giving vent to them. This trait, or characteristic, is sometimes labelled *Type C behaviour* and has been linked to a number of negative health outcomes. For instance, Greer and Morris (1975) found that women with breast cancer demonstrated higher levels of suppressed anger than those with benign tumours, and Grosarth-Maticek *et al.* (1982a) found that emotional suppression was a significant predictor of cancer in two large prospective studies of women who were followed longitudinally.

Determining causality

One of the problems inherent in interpreting the relationship between personality and the onset of disease is that of determining the *direction of causality*. For example, in Greer and Morris's (1975) study of women with breast cancer, it is impossible to know whether the suppressed anger caused the breast cancer or whether the cancer led to emotional suppression as a subsequent coping response.

This 'what comes first, the chicken or the egg?' dilemma is common in health research. However, it can be partially resolved by the use of *prospective studies*, where baseline measures of personality are taken in healthy individuals *before* any evidence of disease is detected. Using this methodology, it is possible to make some assumptions about whether or not the presence, or absence, of certain personality traits has influenced the likelihood of contracting a given disease. For example, as Grosarth-Maticek *et al.*'s (1982) studies were prospective, we could be reasonably confident that the emotional suppression preceded the cancer. However, as the research was *correlational* in nature, it would *not* be able to assert that the emotional suppression *caused* the cancer. At best, it would be possible to assert only that it probably made it more likely. Whilst this might appear to be an overly cautious approach, you might like to consider just how many unknown, third factor variables might have contributed to the onset of breast cancer in the women taking part in the latter author's study.

Owing to the multi-factorial nature of many major diseases, researchers have adopted a range of sophisticated *multi-variate* statistical techniques that provide an accurate picture of the relative importance of multiple variables, or factors (such as personality, age, gender, social class, behaviour, genetic factors, etc.), in predicting disease outcomes. Unfortunately, interpreting the results of such analyses is complex and requires an expert knowledge of research methods and statistics. However, it is generally possible to gain a good understanding of research outcomes by reading the verbal reports in the *discussion section* of a research article. In general, though, whatever the investigator's claims, it is worth noting that no single factor, personality included, is likely to be responsible for the onset or outcome of any given disease.

Dealing with individual differences in personality

Despite the flourishing research investigating the links between personality and disease, very little work has been directed towards helping the health professional to deal with traits that are likely to exert a negative effect on the individual's health. Accordingly, you should note that the following suggestions are only indirectly supported by research.

Hostility and aggression

If HO really is a stable personality trait, habitually expressed by certain patients across a wide range of situations, then there is, arguably, little that can be done in the context of relatively short nursing interventions. However, if we apply Scheier and Bridges' (1995) argument that HO may be a trait that is expressed in response to transient, stressful events, then we have more to work on. We learnt, for example, earlier in this text that hostility and aggression often arise because of a sense of frustration, which may be caused when the individual's goals are blocked, and we learnt that anger was often characteristic of the reactive phase that precludes learned helplessness. In short, anger, aggression and hostility are normally a function of frustration in response to blocked goals and a fear of losing control. Given these factors, it is possible to examine whether specific nursing interventions might be compounding the frustration caused by the patient's condition. For example, interventions that exacerbate feelings of dependency, or which are preceded by a lack of information and a sense of helplessness, are likely to increase or evoke a hostile response. Of course, you should, at all costs, avoid the temptation simply to ascribe hostile or difficult behaviour to personality traits, whilst avoiding consideration of the patient's circumstances.

Fatalism and pessimism

A sense of fatalism and pessimism may be counteracted by trying to promote a sense of *self-efficacy* in the patient. This may be achieved by encouraging the patient to play an active role in planning their own care, and by setting agreed goals that are realistically within the patient's grasp. Success is likely to spawn a sense of personal control over events, which may help the patient to feel less fatalistic about short- and long-term outcomes.

Emotional suppression

Although research suggests that chronic or habitual suppression of emotions, such as anger, may be bad for our health, Keinen *et al.* (1992) caution us from drawing rash conclusions from the available research. They point out that we know very little about the relationship between the suppression of emotion and variables, such as frequency and intensity. In an exploratory study, they found that individuals with the best self-reported health experienced anger infrequently, but were able to express it freely when they did. By contrast, those with the worst self-reported health experienced frequent anger, but often felt unable to express it.

It is possible to read lots of things into this. For example, we could hypothesise that experiencing emotions, such as anger, may not be bad for us *per se*, because their occasional expression may lead to desirable changes in others' behaviour. By the reverse token, we might speculate that emotional suppression stifles potential change, so that the things that are frustrating us go unchallenged. The point is, however, that we don't actually know whether these hypotheses are correct. Furthermore, in a clinical context, the absence of emotion in, say, cardiac patients or individuals with mental health problems, may be due to other factors, such as denial or depression or even, simply, a laid-back personality.

Given this, the bottom line must be that each individual's case needs to be assessed on its own merits, with a full exploration of the relevant circumstances and needs and a sensitive awareness of the patient's emotional status.

Summary

The belief that there is a causal link between personality and disease has a long history dating back to the Ancient Greeks. More recently, however, researchers have begun to explore the relationship between a number of specific personality variables and the increased likelihood of disease. Of these variables, the most extensively researched has been Type A behaviour and its links with coronary heart disease. However, inconsistencies in the data emerging from several large and well-conducted studies have led researchers to focus on a particular sub-component of the Type A construct, namely hostility. In addition to this there is evidence that other personality variables, such as pessimism and fatalism and Type C behaviour, or emotional suppression, increase susceptibility to major diseases such as cancer and increase morbidity and mortality in patients who already have a serious illness.

The correlational nature of this research precludes definite conclusions about a causal linkage between these personality variables and disease. Indeed, although a causal link *may* well exist, the role of personality in the aetiology and maintenance of disease needs to be viewed against a backdrop of many other causal variables, such as diet, genetic links, gender, poverty and differences in lifestyle, such as smoking and alcohol use. In short, most, if not all, major diseases are multi-factorial in origin, and personality is but one of many potential variables.

There are no hard and fast rules for handling individual differences in personality in clinical practice, and, as a consequence, individual cases need to be assessed in relation to the patient's particular circumstances. However, in general terms, efforts should be made to avoid nursing actions that increase the likelihood of frustration and anger or which restrict the patient's opportunities for emotional expression.

Chapter 14

Psychological perspectives on pain

Learning outcomes

By the end of this chapter you should be able to:

- Describe the nature and function of pain.
- Describe the gate theory of pain.
- Summarise the psychological factors that have been shown to affect individual perception of pain.

The nature and function of pain

Pain is an aversive sensory and emotional experience that is usually, though not necessarily, associated with physical damage to the body's tissues. It may be experienced as a dull ache, sharp and stabbing, throbbing and itching or as a burning sensation. Whilst pain is a normal and common phenomenon occurring throughout life, Karoly (1985) points out that it is the most pervasive symptom found in medical practice and is the most common reason why individuals seek medical advice.

There are two main types of pain: *organic*, which results from tissue damage, and *psychogenic*, which is experienced in the absence of any detectable physical damage and which is assumed to be psychological in origin. The distinction between the physical and psychological causes of pain is often blurred (Horn and Munafó 1997). For example, high levels of anxiety or sheer boredom can increase the individual's experience of pain, and psychological disorders such as depression can occasionally result in the experience of moderate to severe pain that appears to be wholly psychological in origin. From a nursing perspective, the rule of thumb should always be that 'pain is what the patient says it is', and certainly, as Bakal (1979) suggests, psychogenic pain should not be automatically dismissed as imaginary simply because no obvious physical aetiology can be found.

Pain is often further sub-divided into *acute* and *chronic*. The former is, by definition, short lasting and subsides as the underlying condition improves. For example, pain resulting from surgical trauma to the surrounding tissues normally decreases as the damaged area heals over time. Chronic pain, however, may persist over many months or years and is associated with intermittent and recurrent conditions such as migraine headaches and neuralgia (a painful inflammation of nerve endings), and with progressive conditions such as rheumatoid arthritis and cancer (Chapman and Bronica 1985). Furthermore, chronic pain (as may be caused by spinal problems) often varies in its intensity, and sufferers may experience relatively pain-free periods interspersed with enduring episodes of severe pain.

Over a longer period of time, the experience of chronic pain can lead to a sense of helplessness or hopelessness and depression, as the patient realises that medical intervention is unable to provide a cure (Boston *et al.* 1990; Anderson *et al.* 1995). The nature of the pain and its debilitating effects can cause the individual to focus further on their condition and the incumbent pain. For example, necessitated restrictions in levels of activity and alcohol intake may lead patients to feel that their social life has been severely curtailed, and the resultant feelings of depression, irritability or aggressive behaviour may cause all but the closest family to withdraw from social interactions with them. Hence, over time, chronic pain can come to dominate individuals' lives and they may come to adopt the sick role (Fordyce and Steger 1979).

Psychogenic pain

According to Sarrafino (1994), there are three basic types of psychogenic pain:

Neuralgia is characterised by a stabbing pain along the course of the nerve (i.e. down one side of the face in facial neuralgia). With this condition, the associated pain is often intermittent and idiosyncratic, in that gentle stimulation with a cotton thread may evoke it, whilst pricking with a needle may not.

Causal neuralgia is characterised by a severe burning pain that occurs at the site of an old wound, sometimes many years after it has healed. The frequency and intensity of the pain may actually increase over time and may encompass other parts of the body.

Phantom limb is often characterised by moderate to intense pain occurring at the site of an amputated limb or some other body part. Patients may, for example, report that they can feel or even move the toes on their amputated foot and they may also experience pain, even when the corresponding nerves have been destroyed. In about 5–10 per cent of cases, the pain associated with phantom limb gets worse over time (Bakal 1979).

It is important to note that, whilst these three types of psychogenic pain all have physical antecedents, purely *psychological events* may be sufficient to evoke physical pain in the absence of any obvious physical cause. For example, Carr (1982, p. 232) notes that the intense grief present in bereavement can cause "feelings of tightness in the throat, choking with shortness of breath and intense subjective distress described as tension or psychological pain".

Models of pain

Specificity and pattern theories of pain

During the 1950s, research into the nature and causes of pain was dominated by two mechanistic models that largely excluded psychological factors as precipitants or contributors to the experience of pain.

According to *specificity theory*, the brain has a specific sensory system that is dedicated to detecting and interpreting pain. Signals sent from pain receptors at various locations in the body are sent to particular regions of the brain where they are processed and recognised as pain. However, according to *pattern theory* there is no separate pain system and the receptors that respond to pain also detect changes in pressure, heat and cold. The theory proposes that these different stimuli yield readily distinguishable patterns that are subsequently interpreted by the brain as touch, pain, etc.

Melzack and Wall (1982) state that neither theory adequately explains the nature of pain. For example, supporters of specificity theory have failed to identify specific pain receptors that do not share sensory information, and no specific region of the brain has been shown to process information about pain. Similarly, pattern theory cannot account for conditions such as neuralgia, where pain can seemingly be evoked by gentle pressure. In addition, neither theory can account for the role of psychological factors in pain perception, nor explain why, for example, negative mood states increase the experience of pain, nor why hypnosis decreases it (Hilgard and Hilgard 1983).

The gate theory of pain

In response to the weaknesses inherent in mechanistic models of pain, Melzack and Wall (1965; 1982) developed the *gate theory of pain*, in an attempt to explain how physiological and psychological factors may act directly to influence the experience of pain. According to the basic theory, a *gating mechanism* (which may be likened to a synaptic cleft

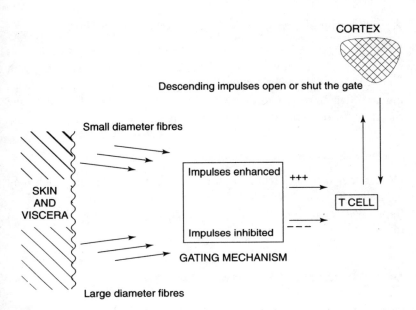

FIGURE 14.1 Schematic diagram of the gate theory of pain

where neural impulses are either inhibited or enhanced) located within the *substantia gelatinosa* (a bundle of nerves that run along the length of the spinal cord) receives signals from peripheral nerve sites via *pain fibres* that have the effect of opening or shutting the gate in varying degrees. Impulses that get through the gate are sent to T or *transmission cells*, which pass *ascending messages* to the brain, where they are experienced as pain. Importantly, however, T cells also receive *descending messages* from the brain, which can also have the effect of inhibiting or enhancing activity at the gate.

Figure 14.1 illustrates the theory schematically, the operation of which may be encapsulated by focusing on the interaction between three basic components, as follows:

1. The amount of activity in the small pain fibres

Small diameter (A delta and C) fibres respond to noxious stimulation at peripheral pain receptor sites. Activity in these small fibres has the effect of opening the gate. The more noxious the stimuli, the more active the fibres and the greater the likelihood of transmission to the T cells and on to the brain where the stimulus is experienced as pain.

2. The amount of activity in the large peripheral pain fibres

Large diameter (A beta) fibres respond to benign stimulation, such as mild irritation, tickling or scratching at peripheral sites. Activity in these fibres has the effect of closing the gate. So, for example, massaging an inflamed or tender area would activate the large fibres and have the effect of reducing the experience of pain.

3. Descending messages from the brain

Descending messages from the brain are sent to the gate, which may have the effect of *either* inhibiting or activating the gating mechanism. As we will learn shortly, both physiological and psychological factors influence pain via this pathway.

Factors affecting pain perception

Endogenous opioids

During the 1800s, the powerful narcotic and analgesic substance *morphine* was identified as the active ingredient of opium, an oriental drug that had been used as a painkiller for hundreds of years. Subsequent research by Hughes *et al.* (1975) revealed the presence of natural or *endogenous opioids* in the body that occur in response to sustained shock or trauma. These substances appear to originate in areas of the mid-brain and in the peripheral nervous system. Furthermore, Horn and Munafó (1997) state that the release of endogenous opioids in the mid-brain has been shown to suppress T cell activity, providing evidence of descending pain inhibition as predicted by the gate theory.

This opioid system can act synergistically with other analgesic mechanisms. For example, simultaneous stimulation of both A delta and A beta fibres inhibits C fibre activity (resulting from dull throbbing pain), and Horn and Munafó state that acupuncture has been shown to produce its analgesic effect by both stimulation of A delta and beta fibres and the release of endogenous opioids.

Neural plasticity and pain memory

There is evidence that damage to tissue can result in *hyperalgesia*, or hypersensitivity to pain, and even resistance to the analgesic effects of powerful painkillers, such as morphine (Woolf 1983; Dubner and Ruda 1992). Why this should occur is unclear. However, Horn and Munafó (1997) suggest that it may be precipitated by *structural changes* in pain neurones and/or disequilibrium in the normal *regulatory balance* maintained by the large and small pain fibres (it is easy to envisage how this might occur as a result of tissue destruction). Such mechanisms may also offer a physiological explanation for pathological pain, such as neuralgia and phantom limb, which can occur long after tissue damage is sustained.

Horn and Munafó (1997) also note that phantom limb is less likely to occur when pain is *inadequately controlled* prior to surgical amputation. They suggest that this should lead us to view pain as an active system that may involve memory-like structures or processes, rather than a passive stimulus-response mechanism. It is certainly an issue that warrants further clinical research.

Anxiety and depression

Pain perception can be negatively influenced by *mood state*, and it is known that anxiety and depression generally exacerbate the experience of pain. Anxiety tends to increase pain only when the anxiety or fear is pain-specific (Dougher *et al.* 1987). For example, anticipatory anxiety may develop in response to repetitive, painful procedures, such as debridement and cleansing of tissue damaged by burning, and Horn and Munafó (1997) draw attention to the possibility that classically conditioned fear reactions might be triggered by such procedures.

Self-focused attention has been shown to increase the subjective experience of mood states (Scheier 1976), and as people with depression often ruminate frequently, this may be one of the mechanisms through which depression alters pain perception. The effects of attentional processes on pain perception are apparent to us all. You may recall, for example, experiencing a significant worsening of toothache, earache or stomach ache as a child or adult as you lay in bed at night with little alternative stimuli to occupy attentional processes. In addition, however, Turk and Fernandez (1991) note that depressed people are also more likely to attribute a *negative meaning* to their pain (i.e. believe that it is due to some underlying fatal condition or some form of punishment for wrong doing, etc.).

As you might have anticipated, pain is also exacerbated by a *perceived loss of control*, and Carr (1982) notes that the pain experienced by terminally ill cancer patients may be relieved through appropriate support, practical help and good communication, all of which are generally regarded as enhancing feelings of control.

Table 14.1 provides a broad overview of types of physical and psychological factors that are likely to influence pain perception.

TABLE 14.1 Physical and psychological factors influencing pain perception

Excitatory factors	Inhibitory factors
Trauma to tissue	Analgesia and counter-stimulation (i.e. massage and acupuncture)
Anxiety and depression, perceived loss of control	Positive coping mechanisms, perceived control
Self-focused attention and negative causal attributions	Diversive activities, externally focused attention
Inappropriate activity	Relaxation, rest, appropriate exercise

Interpretation of pain and personal expectations

Pain is a protective mechanism that alerts us to possible or actual physical damage to the body's systems. Thus, under normal circumstances, pain is interpreted negatively. However, Beecher (1956) showed that soldiers wounded in combat rated their pain as less severe and required less medication than their civilian counterparts with similarly matched wounds. It was suggested that this was due to a positive interpretation of the injuries, owing to the fact that bad wounds often led to soldiers being relieved of duty and returned home. Similarly, there is evidence that pain may be exacerbated through classical conditioning when it is paired with a traumatic event (Sarrafino 1994).

As a consequence, when the patient is faced with a similar event, for a second or third time, he or she may *expect* to experience pain. By the reverse token, however, expectations can also reduce pain. For example, placebos (such as sugar pills administered in place of analgesics) have been shown to reduce reported levels of pain (Melzack and Wall 1982). Placebos are assumed to work because the patient has learnt that analgesics relieve pain, though interestingly enough, there is evidence that they can actually trigger the release of natural *endogenous opiates* in the body (Fields and Levine 1984; Bandura *et al.* 1987).

As mentioned earlier, these substances are naturally produced opiate-like substances, which are released by the body in response to major trauma or sustained physical exertion. In fact, the reason why man-made analgesics such as *morphine* work is because they occupy naturally occurring receptor sites located in the brain and peripheries of the central nervous system (Horn and Munafó 1997). However, endogenous opioids lack the negative side effects of *respiratory depression* and *dependence* associated with their synthetic counterparts.

Psychological treatments for chronic pain

When the patient experiences chronic pain, his or her world may 'shrink', as normal social activities are inhibited and the pain, and its causes, comes to dominate the patient's existence. Under such circumstances, the patient may adopt the *sick role*, which involves inhibition of normal social behaviour and the adoption of abnormal, *pain behaviours*, which may include physical inactivity, heavy reliance on analgesics and decreased autonomy. According to Fordyce (1976), pain behaviour may be positively reinforced by others' responses and by institutional factors. Flor *et al.* (1987), for example, showed that patients' pain behaviour tended to increase when their spouses were attentive to the pain, and Gill *et al.* (1988) demonstrated that children suffering from chronic skin disorders were observed to scratch more when their parents were attentive to the scratching. In addition, pain behaviours may be reinforced by internal factors. For example, inactivity may be linked to a fear (and sometimes also the erroneous belief) that exercise will exacerbate pain.

During the past decade, clinicians and researchers have sought to provide ways of treating pain by focusing on two principal types of intervention: the first concentrating on relieving the muscle tension that exacerbates pain, and the second focusing on individuals' beliefs and perceptions and the pain behaviours that are often incumbent.

(Other methods, including biofeedback and hypnosis, are beyond the scope of this text, but see Horne and Munafó [1997] for a discussion of these treatments.)

Relaxation therapy

Pain can be successfully relieved by the use of *progressive relaxation* methods such as the Jacobsen technique (Jacobsen 1983). This approach involves systematically tensing and relaxing groups of muscles, and works by relieving tension in the whole body or at targeted sites. The rationale behind relaxation training is quite simple. Pain can be generated by muscle tension alone (as, for example, in neck ache or headaches), and therefore relief of muscle tension is also likely to reduce pain caused by specific chronic conditions that affect the skeleto-muscular system (Horne and Munafó 1997). In addition, we now know that counter-stimulation, such as massage, stimulates large, A beta fibre activity, which inhibits pain transmission.

It is important to note that certain conditions, such as arthritis, do not lend themselves to progressive tensioning, and so for such conditions relaxation of muscles and alternative methods, such as the *autogenic method* (Luthe and Schultz 1969), which focuses on the relationship between general tension and breathing, may be more appropriate. Finally, it is worth noting that all methods of relaxation tend to boost the individual's sense of control over the pain, which has both physical and psychological benefits.

Behavioural-cognitive therapy

Fordyce (1976) argued that patients with chronic pain sometimes acquire maladaptive pain behaviours that are reinforced by *secondary gains*, such as an increase in others' attentions and a diminution of personal responsibility. In accordance, behavioural treatments are often aimed at *reshaping behaviour*, by replacing pain behaviours with socially interactive 'well behaviours' that are reinforced by praise, attention and general encouragement.

More recently, this approach has been combined with an increased focus on the self-perceptions, health beliefs and faulty thinking that often underpin chronic pain behaviours. Turk and Fernandez

(1991), for example, have suggested that treatment for cancer pain might include reshaping of maladaptive behaviours by examination and alteration of *negative self-statements* and *erroneous beliefs*. In addition, patients may be encouraged to explore their feelings of helplessness, which are often attributed to the belief that their pain is uncontrollable. These beliefs are challenged (for example, by providing patients with information about the gate control theory) and the patient is encouraged to think more positively, in conjunction with combined behavioural targets set by the therapist.

Choosing the right intervention

A number of evaluation programmes have attempted to establish which treatment approach is most effective, and the results have been inconclusive. It has been argued, for example, that relaxation therapy is the most cost-effective form of pain relief, but some doubt has been cast on its long-term viability as a means of changing chronic pain behaviours (Sarrafino 1994).

As a nurse, you are unlikely to have the time to develop, or put into action, cognitive-behavioural therapies (unless you work in a specialist pain clinic or some similar environment), but you will be able to use some of the basic techniques, such as positive reinforcement and the setting of achievable goals, to help discourage the adoption of the sick role in hospitalised patients. Relaxation techniques, however, are simple to learn and simple to use and may be of considerable benefit in relieving both pain and anxiety in clinical settings, such as palliative or post-surgical care, and they can be taught to psychiatric patients who are excessively anxious.

In addition to the above treatments, you can help to relieve pain by providing the patient with a sense of control. This can be facilitated by supplying the patient with appropriate information about pain and pain relief methods, and by allowing the patient to control the administration of his or her own analgesics where it is appropriate do so. Finally, simple diversion activities can also help to relieve pain. For example, play may be used to distract children's attention away from pain. In short, there is much that can be done to alleviate pain through basic nursing interventions.

Summary

Research into stress, immunology and pain has shown that psychological factors can exert a significant influence over the body's physical systems. Chronic stress can lead to general wear and tear in the cardiac system, impaired immunocompetence and pathological disease states or even death from exhaustion in extreme cases.

Despite the available evidence, it is difficult to determine the extent of the role that stress plays in inducing pathological states in humans. Third factor variables, such as age, gender, genetic factors, lifestyle and personality, also play a role in the aetiology of disease, and in some cases it is not clear whether stress is a result of disease or the cause of it.

Personality variables, such as Type A behaviour, pessimism and fatalism and Type C behaviour, have been shown to have a negative effect on morbidity and mortality, and these can best be handled by examining the situational variables that contribute to such behaviours.

Pain appears to be directly affected by a number of psychological factors that include personal control, mood states, self-focused attention, personal expectations and positive reinforcement. It is hypothesised that these factors influence pain perception by sending inhibitory or excitatory signals to a gating mechanism located in the substantia gelatinosa within the spinal cord.

Providing the patient with information, support and practical help appears to lessen pain perception, possibly by increasing the patient's perception of control and by lessening or preventing anxiety and depression.

MINI SELF-TEST

1   Describe the three phases of the general adaptation syndrome.

2   Describe how stress may impair immunocompetence and lead to disease.

3   Briefly outline the three components that comprise Type A behaviour.

4   Describe what is meant by a third factor variable.

5   Briefly describe organic and psychogenic pain.

6   Outline the failings of the specificity and pattern theories of pain.

7   From memory attempt to draw a diagram of the gate theory of pain.

8   Outline the factors that open and shut the gating mechanism.

9   Describe the main psychological factors that influence pain perception.

10   Outline how pain can be alleviated in clinical practice.

━━━━━━━━━━━━━━━━━━━━━━━━━━━━━ **REFLECTIVE SCENARIOS**

Rosa

Rosa has been suffering from low-grade symptoms of flu and eczema for about twelve months. Things have not been going well at work and she recently split up with her partner.

Briefly explain the possible reasons for her symptoms with reference to the general adaptation syndrome.

Elisabeth

Elisabeth is an 80-year-old woman of Polish descent. She came to the United Kingdom as a refugee during the Second World War and settled after marrying an English man, Bill. He now has advanced Alzheimer's disease and is cared for in a special psychiatric unit located 20 miles from her home. She is finding it increasingly difficult to visit him and is highly distressed by the deterioration in his condition. Furthermore, she feels isolated and lonely as all of her friends have now passed away.

Discuss the risk of Elisabeth developing major disease with reference to stress and immunocompetence and social support.

Alice

Alice is a 32-year-old woman whose mother died of breast cancer. She has recently read an article in a magazine that stated that suppressing anger can significantly heighten the risk of cancer. She is very anxious and describes herself as being unable to express any emotion openly.

Discuss how you might respond to Alice with reference to emotional suppression.

Mark

Mark is a hard-working stockbroker who has recently been diagnosed as having hypertension. An interview with his doctor reveals that he has a family history of heart disease. In addition, he smokes and drinks heavily and admits to feeling under intense pressure to maximise profits day in day out and to getting bad tempered and irritable when under pressure.

Discuss whether Mark is at increased risk of developing coronary heart disease at some point in the future with reference to Type A behaviour.

Said

Said has rheumatoid arthritis and has learned that the pain he experiences is often worse when he is low in mood or worried.

Explain this phenomenon with reference to the gate theory of pain and concepts such as self-focused attention and mood.

Lena

Lena is awaiting surgery for cancer of the throat. She is openly anxious about being disfigured and about the effect it may have on her marriage. She also expresses concern about not being able to cope with the pain following her operation.

Discuss how Lena's anxiety about disfigurement and her fear of rejection may contribute to the pain that she is likely to experience post-operatively.

Hanna

Hanna is a 50-year-old woman who suffers from intermittent facial neuralgia that causes her considerable distress and pain. She tells you that she sometimes gets the impression that her doctor thinks her problem is largely psychological in origin.

Using your knowledge of pain theory and concepts such as neural plasticity, pain-memory and anxiety, describe how you might provide Hanna with an explanation for her condition.

Tom

Tom is an 8-year-old who suffers from haemophilia. He has been receiving orthopaedic treatment for a ligament problem, which has necessitated the use of callipers to support both legs. Tom frequently experiences pain, and the staff have become concerned that he is becoming over-reliant on powerful analgesics, such as pethidine hydrochloride.

Discuss how you might conceivably seek to reduce his reliance on painkillers, with reference to concepts such as pain behaviours, positive reinforcement and reshaping behaviour.

Suggested reading

Horn, S. and Munafó, M. (1997). *Pain: Theory research and intervention.* Buckingham: Open University Press.
This book provides a rich and authoritative source of information about pain, its causes, mechanisms and treatments. It may be particularly useful for students carrying out advanced project work on pain.

Sarrafino, E. P. (1994). *Health Psychology: Biopsychosocial interactions.* New York: John Wiley and Sons.
This informative text provides an excellent overview of the topic of stress set in a health context.

Simmons, M. and Daw, P. (1994). *Stress, Anxiety and Depression: A practical workbook.* Bicester: Winslow Press.
As the title suggests, this is very much a practical, down-to-earth text that provides interesting reading and is aimed at showing how stress, anxiety and depression can be effectively managed.

Part five

Applying psychological knowledge in clinical practice

Chapter 15

Building and applying a psychological framework in clinical practice

Learning outcomes

By the end of this chapter you should be able to:

- Describe what a hypothesis is.
- Understand how hypothesis formulation can be used to guide nursing actions.
- Describe how functional analysis can be used to generate a hypothesis.

Applying psychological knowledge in clinical practice

We have now reached the final section of this book and will turn our attention to how psychological knowledge may be used in clinical practice. The aim is to demonstrate how your knowledge base can be used to form and test hypotheses that may be used to guide your actions in clinical situations. In doing so, we will also briefly explore how knowledge is translated into a meaningful, conceptual framework.

It is important to note that we will be concerned only with psychological problems and needs in this section, although many, if not all, of the ideas and concepts discussed could be applied equally to the identification and assessment of physical and social problems.

Assessment and hypothesis formulation

Accurate identification of the individual's problems and needs is critical to the process of effective nursing care, as it determines both the relevance and quality of the nursing actions that follow. (This can be directly equated with our use of the concepts of understanding and reflection in the first chapter.) Identification of problems and needs is often straightforward and relies on verbal reports obtained directly from the patient or client. From time to time, however, instances occur where sufficient information cannot be obtained from verbal reports alone, and the nurse must use clinical judgement to combine information from other sources, such as observation and case history, with his or her knowledge base and experience to piece together a picture of the problems inherent in the situation. In effect, the nurse reaches an assumption or conclusion about what may be happening and this *inferential process* is called *hypothesis formulation*.

Forming a hypothesis by extrapolating from information available in the situation can benefit the individual concerned. The health professional's expert level of knowledge and experience can lead to insights into the patient's world that facilitate an understanding of what *is* happening or a prediction of what *may* happen at some future point in time, given the individual's emotional state and particular circumstances.

Although the term 'hypothesis' sounds rather complex and technical, it may be defined simply as 'a supposition used as a basis from which to draw conclusions' (Collins English Dictionary). Furthermore, you may be surprised to learn that nurses frequently generate and apply hypotheses, though few would actually use this term to describe this type of clinical judgement. An experienced nurse, for example, admitting an elderly patient who is mentally confused, may observe the dryness of his skin, gain information from his wife that suggests the change in his condition was rapid with no preceding evidence of infection or trauma, and so draw the conclusion that the patient has a toxic confusional state, caused by dehydration. Having made this judgement, she would probably seek medical confirmation of her hypothesis, rehydrate the patient and wait to observe a consequent improvement in his condition.

This is not an exacting experimental process as a scientist would know it, simply because the validity of the nurse's hypothesis cannot be rigorously tested within the constraints of the human and clinical context. When dealing with the individual, the nurse has no access to a control group and she cannot attempt to *disconfirm* her hypothesis by waiting to see if the patient's mental state deteriorates further without rehydration. Nevertheless, the hypothesis is more than a simple guess or hunch. It is an assumption or conclusion based on the accumulation of knowledge and experience, and the nurse seeks to verify the hypothesis by instigating appropriate nursing actions designed to change and improve the patient's condition. If these actions fail to result in improvement, the nurse will generate a new hypothesis, leading to a new course of action and so on, until a valid hypothesis finally results in improvement in the patient's condition.

One very important function of hypothesis generation is to *raise awareness* of potential problems. So even if no formal nursing action is taken at an early stage, the resulting anticipation or awareness of issues leads to a heightened sensitivity to cues that might indicate the development of the anticipated problem or problems. This is an essential element of reflective practice, which draws on the nurse's knowledge, experience, observation skills and problem-solving skills.

The generation of a hypothesis sometimes involves multidisciplinary inputs, which may be brought together in case conferences as the following case study shows. This study, based in a psychiatric setting, provides an illustration of why hypothesis formulation is necessary when a patient is unwilling or simply unable to provide information about the nature and cause of their problems. The name of the individual concerned has been changed for reasons of confidentiality.

Carol

Carol had suffered from an obsessive-compulsive (OC) disorder, which had necessitated several admissions to an acute psychiatric hospital over a period of years. She often experienced high levels of anxiety which, as is often the case with OC disorders, could only be relieved by performing a ritualistic act. In her case, this led to an irresistible urge to cleanse herself; as a consequence, when she got really anxious, she would shower up to two to three times an hour and continually wash her clothes, so being unable to leave the vicinity of the bathroom. On past occasions, admission to hospital had always resulted in a marked decline in ritualistic behaviour, and she would return home within a few weeks (the ritualistic behaviour was still present, but at acceptable levels that did not interfere grossly with her daily life). On this particular occasion, however, her behaviour had spiralled out of control, and after many weeks on the acute unit there was still no sign of an improvement.

Given her past history and the divergence from the normal pattern of short admission and discharge, a case conference was called to try and ascertain what was causing or contributing to her current behaviour. In effect, the team assembled to formulate a hypothesis that might lead to an effective course of action.

As Carol did not feel able to discuss details of her situation, the team explored her case history in detail, in an effort to find clues about the causes of her behaviour. The team worked initially on the widely accepted hypothesis that OC acts serve to relieve anxiety, and as the frequency of the acts had significantly increased, the team deduced that something must have been causing her intense anxiety. At this point, one of the key workers, who had known Carol over a period of years, told the team that Carol had always had a rocky and fractious relationship with her husband, who had great difficulty dealing with her obsessive behaviour. She added that she suspected Carol no longer loved her husband and secretly longed to get out of the relationship, but that she could not contemplate divorce or separation, because of her strict religious background and sense of duty. It was thus hypothesised further that their relationship had reached a critical point and that Carol's behaviour was a way of (unconsciously) saying that she could no longer cope. It was also noted that, in one of very few discourses, Carol had indicated that she might consider going to a half-way house or hostel rather than go home. This led to a further shaping of the original hypothesis on the basis that her illness and behaviour might be a way of effectively ending her marriage without experiencing feelings of excessive guilt (there is a moral and legal argument that you cannot be held responsible for your actions if you are mentally disturbed).

The team were reluctant to sanction this option, because it was felt that she could become permanently institutionalised in long-term psychiatric care. However, the alternatives were to allow her to remain on the acute admissions unit, which was not desirable or viable in the longer term, or to send her home again. In consideration of this latter option, the team noted that if their hypothesis was right and Carol's behaviour was a way of avoiding an intolerable marital situation, then sending her home might result in a catastrophic sequence of events. As a consequence, the team agreed to investigate whether a suitable placement could be found for her in a hostel or home with supervision.

Although the latter example draws on a case study based in psychiatric practice, it could just as easily have involved hypothesis formulation when the question centered on whether a child should be returned to a parent with a drugs problem or it could have involved a discussion ensuing during a handover about whether a patient should be told he had cancer, given that his wife did not want him to know. Indeed, as the scenario illustrates, the use of hypothesis formulation as an 'educated guess ' is particularly useful when the patient or client lacks insight into their condition, as may occur, for example, when the individual is a young child, a confused, severely depressed or deluded patient or when the patient is simply unwilling, for whatever reason, to discuss their situation.

Testing a hypothesis

An important element in the process of constructing a *working hypothesis* is the inclusion of some form of check that the nursing actions that flow from it result in an improvement or resolution of a particular problem or problems. This is called *hypothesis testing*, and in Carol's case the team expected and, indeed, found a reduction in the frequency of showering activity after she was told that she would soon be transferred to a hostel or home, which served to confirm the hypothesis that her behaviour was an unconscious way of seeking an exit from her marriage that would avoid overwhelming feelings of guilt.

Sometimes a formal baseline of behaviour may be established in order to assess whether or not a hypothesis is valid. In Carol's case, this information was readily available in the nursing notes, so an average or approximation of her showering behaviour (i.e. how many showers per day) was used to establish a baseline, against which subsequent behaviour was compared. However, in many instances it is more practical and desirable to test a hypothesis informally. Say, for example, that in working with a burns patient your hypothesis is 'she has a low self-esteem' and you decide 'I'll make sure I give her regular attention and try to boost her confidence levels when I can'. Given the situation, it would be impractical, and arguably unhelpful, to make a formal assessment of her level of self-esteem, and it would be better simply to observe whether or not her mood lifted over a period of time. Of course, you could not be sure that any improvement in mood was due to your actions, but this would be relatively unimportant. In fact, formal baselines of assessment are more typically used when some form of 'expert intervention' or formal programme of care is instituted by the likes of a psychologist or psychiatrist, though nurses may still be actively involved in this process. For example, you might be asked to monitor and formally record changes in eating behaviour in a young child being treated for a choking phobia, or you might be asked to record the frequency of aggressive incidents in a teenager with severe learning disabilities and behavioural problems.

Using a functional analysis to generate a working hypothesis

Functional analysis is a useful and relatively straightforward technique that can be used to assess the causes and consequences of behaviour, which may, in turn, be used to help generate a working hypothesis or hypotheses. This technique, sometimes referred to as the *ABC of behaviour*, comprises three basic stages of analysis (Herbert 1996):

B the behaviour(s)

First, details of the *target behaviour* are noted. The details depend on the clinical context, but typically involve documenting what the behaviour is, how often it occurs, where and when it occurs and how intense it is. For example, a health visitor following up a mother's anxiety about a recurrence of bed-wetting in her 4-year-old son might want to ascertain when the problem started, how much urine was being passed and how many times a night it occurred and when.

A the antecedent(s)

Next, details of events or stimuli preceding the target behaviour are noted and retained or eliminated as possible causes or contributing factors. So the health visitor might, for example, ask what he drank prior to going to bed, whether there was any change in his usual routine, whether there was anything of particular note happening at home, or whether there were any symptoms that might indicate the presence of a urinary tract infection.

C the consequences

Finally, the health visitor would seek information about the possible consequences of the target behaviour, on the basis, for example, that the parent's response might actually serve to *reinforce* the behaviour or make it more likely to recur. (This approach is based on Thorndike's *law of effect* [1898], which states that behaviour is modified by its consequences. At its most simple, behaviour that has positive consequences is likely to repeated, whilst that which has negative consequence is not).

Using the information gleaned from this technique, the health visitor would start to piece together a picture of what was happening, leading to the generation of a hypothesis and subsequent suggestions for action to resolve the problem. She might, for example, discover that the child was wetting the bed once a night, two or three times a week, and that there was no evidence of infection or obvious change in his personal routine (like drinking more than usual prior to going to bed). She might then look for other possible antecedents and discover that the boy was worried about starting school and had frequent wakings during the night that were *not* accompanied by bed wetting. She might, therefore, hypothesise that the cause of bed-wetting was linked to anxiety about starting school and she might then ask the parents how they reacted when he wet the bed. She might discover that they were fairly calm and relaxed about it and that they were doing nothing that would inadvertently reinforce his behaviour. As a consequence, she might simply suggest to the parents that, with patience, the problem would decline and encourage them to talk to their son about schooling and to offer reassurance where appropriate.

Using a knowledge base to generate hypotheses

Nurses frequently use their knowledge and experience to formulate hypotheses. A nurse in charge of a casualty unit, for example, may discharge a patient with the instructions 'contact us if there are any further problems or if you experience x, y and z', only to receive a phone call a few hours later describing some of the symptoms and being asked 'do you think it's serious and should I come back?' Similarly, a community-based midwife may have to decide whether a mother's symptoms warrant urgent hospitalisation or not, and a health visitor may be asked whether a child's continued 'colic' might actually be a symptom of a viral infection or some other underlying pathology. In each case, the nurse draws on his or her knowledge base, experience and a modicum of common sense to formulate a hypothesis and decide on an appropriate course of action.

Benner (1984) argues that, given sufficient experience, nurses reach conclusions about the appropriate course of action in clinical situations so readily that the whole process is characterised by a degree of automaticity or a simple, intuitive, 'knowing' what has to be done. (Though Benner notes that this automaticity is quickly lost when the situation is novel, unusual or particularly complex.) Conway *et al.* (1998) suggest that such *knowing behaviour* is underpinned by, or is characteristic of, the development of a conceptual or schematic framework that organises information in a meaningful way, so as to allow ready access to relevant facts, memories and experiences in a given context (in much the same way that a library indexing system allows you access to thousands of books that would otherwise be unobtainable without some form of organising system). When knowledge is consolidated in this way, the individual is able to make rapid decisions that have an intuitive feel. By the reverse token, however, the novice student must gradually build a conceptual framework from raw knowledge and 'hands-on' experience by following rules, recalling events and incidents and by applying facts to the situation in a deterministic and mechanical way. Dreyfus and Dreyfus (1996) liken this to the process involved in learning to drive a car. At first your actions are mechanical and you have to think consciously through each step – checking the mirror, using the clutch, selecting a gear, pulling away from the kerb, etc. – and the whole process soaks up reserves of attentional capacity. After a while, however, the task is less consuming, and as you get more proficient you are able to think ahead, anticipate what other drivers are up to and simultaneously hold a conversation with a friend, because you simply *know* what to do.

So how does this relate to you as a student? Well first of all, when you start learning to apply psychology in clinical settings, you will not have access to a fully developed conceptual framework and you will not simply 'know what to do'. Instead, when faced with a problem, you are likely to find yourself consciously sifting and sorting though bits of information to form a hypothesis. (This is no bad thing and something that even experts ought to do more often!) Second, given that facts do not exist in a vacuum, but hang together in a way that makes conceptual sense, you are likely to retain only the information that you perceive as being important, whilst discarding that which you regard as being redundant. Furthermore, what you retain as important is likely to be drawn from three principal sources:

- Information or facts that fit with your personal experience (i.e. that link into an existing conceptual schema or schemas).
- Information supplied by the lecturer, colleagues or friends that impresses you with its salience or apparent usefulness.
- Information that is validated at some later point in time through your own personal experiences in and out of clinical practice.

As you progress through your career, the importance of direct personal experience is likely to wield a progressively stronger influence on learning processes and on what information is retained or discarded. An important part of this process will involve generating hypotheses based on your knowledge base and retaining ideas, concepts and theories that seem to work. Of course, faced with so much to learn you may be tempted to discard some material quite early in your course. This inclination is natural enough and may, at times, feel like a necessary self-preservation strategy. However, you need to ask yourself 'how do I know what to retain or discard?' The answer to this is, of course, that you do not, which is why teachers and clinicians are so keen on ensuring that students acquire a broad knowledge base during their programme of training!

In summary, the linkage between theory and practice and the ability to apply psychological knowledge in a meaningful way is a function of reflective practice, which involves testing the validity of nursing actions through the generation and testing of hypotheses.

Using a model to generate hypotheses

Given that psychology is such a complex subject, it can be useful to adopt a model or framework as a means of generating hypotheses about the patient's situation. The choice of model may vary depending on the context of the situation. In the following example, we will adopt Moos' (1982) *adaptive tasks* as a model for generating ideas.

Jenny is a 10-year-old girl who has been admitted to the regional renal unit, following the development of chronic nephritis and renal failure, as a result of an immunologic reaction to infection elsewhere in the body. The plan is to establish a semi-permanent A-V shunt (artery to vein shunt) that will permit hemodialysis, which she will have to undergo several times a week until a suitable transplant donor is found. A minor surgical procedure is required to create the A-V shunt from existing tissue, and it will need to withstand the fairly high levels of pressure necessary to facilitate the exit and return flow of blood from the body to the dialysis machine.

Problem-needs identification and hypothesis formulation

On Jenny's admission to the unit, Gill is appointed as key-worker to work with her and she tries to strike up a rapport. Jenny, however, is quite morose and reticent, which Gill feels is understandable given that she is physically unwell and has found herself in an alien environment with the imminent prospect of major changes occurring in her life. Amy, a third year student nurse, expresses a particular interest in Jenny and asks Gill if she can work closely with her. In particular, she is keen to explore how Jenny is coping emotionally with the situation.

Given that Jenny is reluctant to talk about how she feels, Amy decides to use Moos' adaptive tasks (see p. 59) as a model or framework to generate ideas about the concerns and anxieties that Jenny might have and to try and generate testable, working hypotheses that can be used to guide her care.

Amy uses the model in the following way, considering each of the model's points in turn and applying her knowledge base and common sense to decide which may be relevant in Jenny's case:

Points 1 and 2. Dealing with pain, incapacitation and other symptoms and dealing with the hospital environment and special treatment procedures

Amy thinks that Jenny may well be worried about possible pain and discomfort resulting from the procedure to establish the A-V shunt and about the forthcoming dialysis. She also feels that Jenny may harbour other fears, such as anxiety about the consequences of the dialysis procedure failing. Amy considers these points and combines it with her knowledge of the relationship between psychological factors and pain to formulate the hypothesis that anxiety about the A-V and dialysis procedures is likely to exacerbate any pain and discomfort that Jenny may experience. Amy realises that she cannot directly test this hypothesis, but she decides that her first plan of action should be to try and discover whether Jenny does indeed harbour such fears and to allay them where possible by providing information about pain control and by being alert to any anxieties expressed about forthcoming clinical procedures.

Point 3. Developing and maintaining adequate relationships with health care staff

Amy thinks that Jenny may find it difficult to establish relationships with members of staff and other patients, not least because she is the only child currently being treated on the unit. At first, Amy is unsure how to deal with this, but then she recalls that role modelling can have a positive effect on behaviour. She thinks about involving a specific female patient, who she knows is robust and optimistic in her attitude to dialysis and life in general. Amy forms the hypothesis that as well as serving as a potential friend in a strange environment, the patient might also serve as a positive role model that will help Jenny to deal with the prospect of dialysis. Amy decides to test this by trying to facilitate a relationship between the two and observing the outcome.

Points 4 and 5. Preserving a reasonable emotional balance and preserving a satisfactory self-image

Amy considers this point and recalls that events that threaten major, negative change can result in a crisis or disequilibrium in the self-system. Amy speculates that from Jenny's perspective, the prospect of having an A-V shunt and being linked to a machine for several hours a week could lead to negative changes in body image that might be difficult to reconcile. She therefore forms the hypothesis that Jenny will have emotional difficulty adapting to her new self-image. She decides to test this by encouraging Jenny to talk about how she feels and to observe her non-verbal behaviour for evidence of anxiety. Amy knows that she will have to tread carefully, however. She remembers that individuals sometimes use defence mechanisms, such as denial, to protect themselves when they feel threatened. She also recalls that denial can be adaptive and she does not want to push Jenny into talking about her condition if she is not ready to do so.

Point 6. Preserving a relationship with family and friends

Amy has learnt that social support is an important factor in mediating the individual's response to threatening or challenging events. She knows that Jenny's most important source of social support is her family. However, she has been informed that the family tends to be overprotective and she recalls that learned helplessness can occur if too much is done for individuals in a vulnerable position. She adopts the hypothesis that Jenny's sense of self-efficacy will be boosted by encouraging her to take control of her care programme. Amy is not sure how to test this and realises that she needs to think more carefully about the sort of procedures that Jenny might safely be encouraged to do for herself. So she decides to discuss this further with Gill, but for the time being makes a special note in the care plan that although the team should seek to involve the family in Jenny's treatment, care should be taken to minimise the likelihood of Jenny feeling overwhelmed and out of control.

Point 7. Preparing for an uncertain future

Amy knows that uncertainty due to factors such as lack of information about events that threaten the self is a major and almost universal source of stress, and she also recalls that an individual's appraisal of what an event will mean for them is mediated by the extent to which they believe they can deal with it successfully. She thinks again about role modelling and it reaffirms her belief that finding a positive role model would be a good thing in terms of showing Amy that it is possible to live with dialysis and have a reasonable quality of life. However, she returns to the issue of uncertainty and feels that the core issue is to do with the reduction of stress through the provision of appropriate information. On the basis of this, Amy forms the hypothesis that providing Jenny with information will make the future less uncertain and hence less frightening. She decides to test this by being receptive to any questions, doubts or anxieties that Jenny may have and by gradually providing her with information about the procedures and outcomes. Amy notes that she will closely monitor what effect this has.

A note to end

I chose to adopt Moos' model for this scenario, because I felt it was the most appropriate in the circumstances. I could, however, have chosen an alternative framework or model or I might have elected to construct a care plan without redress to a model at all. In fact, there is no right or wrong way of applying psychological care. There are no definitive truths and only general rules to guide you. In the end, what you choose to do and how you do it will be determined by your personal knowledge and experience and the extent to which you actively engage in reflective thought.

Summary

Accurate assessment of needs and problems is an essential prerequisite to high-quality nursing care. An important assessment tool is the formulation of a working hypothesis that can be tested through the effectiveness of nursing actions. A hypothesis may be used to explain an individual's emotional state or behaviour in an ongoing situation, or it may be used to anticipate or predict events that might feasibly occur given certain circumstances. If the actions that flow from a hypothesis prove to be ineffective in improving the individual's condition, a new hypothesis is generated and the nursing actions that flow from it are again monitored and evaluated. This sequence of events may be repeated until a successful hypothesis results in an improvement in the individual's emotional state or behaviour.

Functional analysis is a technique that may be used to help generate a working hypothesis, by providing the nurse with information about the target behaviour(s), its antecedents and its consequences. Such information can be invaluable in building up a picture of what is happening when individuals are unable or unwilling to provide information themselves.

Psychological models can also be used to generate hypotheses in given clinical situations, and the selection of an appropriate model rests on the judgement of the individual practitioner. The model may be used as a framework for identifying particular problems that might feasibly arise, and the formulation of subsequent hypotheses can prove invaluable, as they encourage the nurse to test the effectiveness of the nursing actions that flow from them.

Over time, your ability to generate hypotheses will improve as your knowledge base grows and as your experience informs you what tends to work and what does not. However, it is important to remember that no two individuals or situations are ever the same, and your need to generate ideas and to test solutions tailored to the individual will be as great in twenty years' time as it is now.

MINI SELF-TEST

1   Briefly outline what is meant by formulating a hypothesis.

2   Why is it sometimes necessary to draw inferences from information available in the situation?

3   How can a functional analysis be used to generate a working hypothesis?

4   Describe what is meant by the statement that novice students must actively construct knowledge.

5   Why do you think a model may be useful for generating hypotheses?

Suggested reading

Benner, P. (1984). *From Novice to Expert: Excellence and power in clinical practice.* Menlo Park: Addison-Wesley.
This is Benner's original text, and although many of her ideas have been subject to criticism, it is well worth reading.

Benner, P. A., Tanner, C. A. and Chelsa, C. A. (1996). *Expertise in Nursing Practice: Caring, clinical judgement and ethics.* New York: Springer Publishing Co.
This up-to-date text elaborates on many of the issues raised in Benner's original text.

The following texts are fairly specialised, but provide a useful starting point for understanding how memories are constructed and applied.

Baddely, A. D. (1982). *Your Memory: A user's guide.* New York: Macmillan Press.

Neisser, U. (Ed.) (1982). *Memory Observed: Remembering in natural contexts.* San Francisco: Freeman Publishing Co.

Tulving, E. (1983). *The Elements of Episodic Memory.* New York: Oxford University Press.

Glossary of psychological and medical terms

Abnormal grief An atypical grief reaction that may involve an absent or prolonged reaction often including chronic feelings of guilt, sadness and anxiety.

Acceptance The final stage in the Kubler-Ross Model of death and dying. It should not be confused with adaptation, wherein the individual may adjust to events rather than accept them.

Acute A term used to describe an event, such as illness or pain, that has a rapid onset and is transient rather than ongoing.

Aetiology The cause of some disease or condition.

Affect A prevailing or enduring mood state such as depression or joviality.

AIDS Short for Acquired Immune Deficiency Syndrome. A disorder that results in an impaired immune response and death from secondary infections or cancers.

Alzheimer's (disease) The leading cause of dementia in elderly people. Normal brain functions are interrupted by the build up of protein-like substances in the brain causing severe disorientation and memory loss.

Anger A strong emotion that is evoked when goals are blocked, occurring especially if the act is viewed as intentional and avoidable.

Anorexia nervosa An eating disorder characterised by perceptual disturbance, marked weight loss and fear of gaining weight.

Antecedent A term meaning that which goes before. For example, chronic stress may be an antecedent of heart disease.

Antibody A term used to describe a type of immune cell that is produced in response to a specific antigen.

Anticipated loss An emotional and cognitive reaction to the threat of loss of a body part, status, someone close or of life itself.

Antigen A term used to describe foreign bodies or pathogens such as bacteria and viruses.

Appendectomy Surgical removal of the appendix.

Attachment An emotional bond between two people.

Attitude An individual's like or dislike of objects, peoples, groups, etc. Often taken to comprise an affective and behavioural component and the individual's beliefs and values.

Attribution The process by which we attribute or apportion blame for events to internal or external sources.

Autism A psychological disorder involving aloofness and flat affect. May be associated with dysfunction in centres of the brain that control social behaviour. Typically first diagnosed from the age of 3.

Autonomic nervous system The division of the peripheral nervous system into the sympathetic and parasympathetic systems. Genetic differences in ANS activity are assumed to influence individual differences in behaviour.

B cell A type of immune response cell that produces specific antibodies that disable pathogens by locking onto their surface and preventing them from replicating.

Bargaining Often seen as a reaction to anticipated loss, the individual attempts to stave off the loss by striking bargains with powerful others, such as doctors in charge of their care.

Barriers to action A term used to describe anything that might prevent an individual seeking help, for example financial barriers, stigmas, personal fear, etc.

Belief in a just world A belief that the world is an ordered and fair place, where good and evil reap their just rewards.

Bereavement A term used to describe the characteristic response exhibited by individuals who have lost someone close.

Bulimia A class of eating disorder that involves a pattern of binge eating and self-induced vomiting. It is sometimes associated with anorexia.

Burnout A chronic stress disorder that is characterised by anger, irritation, impatience, insomnia and depression. It is often found in health workers and is associated with the emotional strain of caring for others over time.

Caesarean section Surgical removal of the neonate through the abdominal wall.

Cannula A small round instrument used for insertion into the body.

Causal neuralgia A type of neuralgia occurring at the site of an old wound that may increase with intensity over time.

Centile A unit of measurement used to assess parameters such as height and weight. For example, a 5-year-old male whose height lay around the 70th centile would have 70 children smaller and 30 taller than him.

Chemotherapy The use of small quantities of toxic agents to fight diseases such as cancer.

Cholesterol A fat or lipid that circulates in the blood stream. It can attach to the walls of the arteries narrowing the lumen, which may result in circulatory problems and heart disease.

Chronic A term used to describe an ongoing event or condition, such as illness or pain.

Chronic sorrow A term used to describe unresolved grief that may last for many years or indefinitely in some cases.

Classical conditioning A theory of learning that holds that novel behaviours occur as a function of repeated stimulus–response associations.

Clinical depression Severe to moderate depression that substantially interferes with the individual's daily life. Sometimes referred to as pathological depression.

Cognitive self-awareness A complex cognitive function that allows the individual to be an object of his or her own knowledge and to plan and reflect on the causes and consequences of one's own and other's behaviour.

Cold cognitions Cognitions that are rational, neutral and non-self-evaluative.

Compartmentalisation A term used to describe the process wherein strong emotions are successfully processed or dealt with following a major event, such as bereavement.

Compliance A term used when a patient follows health advice. The term adherence is preferred by some authors, because it implies less of a patient–practitioner power imbalance.

Conflict theory A model that outlines a characteristic pattern of responses to urgent threats to the individual's well-being.

Confounding A term used to describe the case where an investigator cannot draw conclusions about the relationship between the independent and dependent variables in a study, because of the influence of third factor variables.

Controlled study An experimental study where the investigator has attempted to control, or account for, the effects of third factor variables.

Correlation A mathematical term used to indicate that two or more variables are interlinked. A positive correlation indicates that as one variable increases the other does too, whilst a negative correlation indicates that as one variable increases the other declines.

Cortisol One of the 'stress hormones' produced by the adrenal glands. It is an anti-inflammatory steroid that increases blood glucose and causes water retention.

Costs versus benefits A term borrowed from the study of economics. Used to describe or measure an individual's beliefs about the advantages and disadvantages involved in seeking help or complying with treatment.

Cues to action A term used to describe anything that makes health protective behaviour more likely, for example health campaigns, user-friendly consultation hours, etc.

Debridement A painful clinical procedure, whereby dead or necrotic tissue is removed to allow new growth. It is often necessary in order to promote healing following severe to moderate burns.

Denial A conscious or unconscious denial of reality. Much like illusory self-perceptions, except that denial is more often viewed as a maladaptive defence mechanism.

Dependent variable A term used to describe a variable that is changed in some way by an independent variable or variables in an experimental study. The dependent variable is often a response.

Depersonalisation A feeling that one is little more than an inconsequential number or cog in a large system or machine. It can also refer to a psychiatric condition where the individual feels unreal.

Diabetes mellitus Also referred to as insulin-dependent diabetes. It is caused by a deficiency in insulin synthesis.

Dialysis Treatment of the body's waste products following kidney failure. Peritoneal dialysis is more commonly used in children awaiting transplantation. Hemodialysis is used in conjunction with an A-V shunt, when peritoneal dialysis is contraindicated or when dialysis is expected to be long term.

Diseases of adaptation A group of diseases that are believed to result from exposure to chronic stress, such as hypertension and ulcers.

Downward social comparison A mental defence mechanism wherein the individual compares his or her situation with someone worse off as a means of bolstering self-esteem.

DSM IV Diagnostic and Statistical Manual, version four. One of a series of classification tools that are used to help clinicians make psychiatric diagnoses.

Ecological validity The extent to which a scientific construct has 'real world' value.

Embarrassment An aversive, but transient, response characterised by blushing, a downward gaze and feelings of awkwardness that occur in response to some minor violation of social standards.

Emotional suppression A term sometimes used to describe a habitual tendency to suppress emotions such as anger. The emotions may be internalised, rather than expressed openly.

Endocrine Glands of internal secretion, such as the pancreas or thyroid glands.

Endogenous depression Meaning to arise from within, it is used to describe depression caused by internal, biological events.

Epilepsy A disorder caused by random firing of neurones. There are two primary types: petit mal, which can cause brief lapses of consciousness, and grand mal, which results in major convulsions that can be life-threatening if they occur in rapid succession.

Epinephrine A 'stress hormone' secreted by the adrenal medulla. It raises heart rate and blood pressure and is also known as 'adrenaline'.

External (situational) variables Anything external to the individual that can be used to explain his or her behaviour.

Factor A psychological term often used interchangeably with the term 'variable' . It refers to a thing, dimension or component of some psychological construct. For example, reading skill and problem-solving ability are important factors in the construct 'intelligence'.

Faulty thinking A term used in clinical psychology to describe the negative thinking often seen in individuals who are depressed. Sometimes referred to as a 'depressive set'.

Fear of negative evaluation An intense anticipatory anxiety based on the belief that one's behaviour or character is likely to be judged negatively by others.

Flight–fight response An instinctive response to threats that activates the sympathetic autonomic nervous system in preparation for extraordinary levels of physical activity.

Flooding A treatment for specific phobias that involves immediate and marked exposure of the individual to a feared stimulus, as opposed to a gradual exposure.

Fundamental attribution error A law that states that individuals tend to attribute error in others' behaviour to internal (person) variables.

Gate theory of pain A theory that explains how psychological and physiological factors may influence pain perception. Underpinning the theory is a hypothesised gating mechanism, which mediates pain perception.

Generalised anxiety disorder An enduring state of generalised anxiety that is not linked to specific situational causes.

Global A term used to describe a phenomenon that is pervasive and not localised to specific aspects of self. For example, a global loss of self-esteem typically results from a belief that *every* aspect of self is worthless.

Grief An intense and unique emotional reaction that accompanies bereavement.

Guilt A private emotion that occurs when an individual believes that his or her actions have harmed another and when he or she feels personally responsible and believes that the act could have been avoided.

Haemophilia A disorder, rare in females, that is caused by a lack of Factor VIII, which helps the blood to clot. It is genetically transmitted and results in painful internal bleeding that causes chronic damage to joints and/or potentially fatal blood loss. Is now effectively managed by self-administration of Factor VIII.

Hardiness A personality trait or disposition much like self-efficacy that is characterised by a sense of personal control and commitment.

Health protective behaviour Any behaviour carried out by an individual for the purpose of maintaining health.

Help-seeking behaviour A term used to describe actions that lead the individual to seek (early) help for signs and symptoms of disease.

HO Short for hostility and aggression. A personality trait associated with Type A behaviour and coronary heart disease.

Hot cognitions Thought processes that arise as a function of a personal crisis where the self is threatened.

Hypertension Raised blood pressure. Essential hypertension refers to symptoms of unknown aetiology. May be treated by the use of hypotensive drugs.

Ideal and actual self A psychological construct based on the premise that individuals have an ideal self (linked to personal self-standards) that is sometimes contrasted with the actual self, i.e. as witnessed by our actual behaviour.

Illness schema An internal model or representation of the cause and course of (typically common) illness.

Illusory self-perceptions A term used to describe a phenomenon wherein individuals hold exaggerated and unrealistic beliefs about their abilities, appearance, importance, etc.

Immunocompetence A term used to describe the general effectiveness of the immune system.

Independent variable A term used to describe a variable in an experimental study that has a measurable effect on a dependent variable. For example, in Friedman and Rosenman's study, Type A behaviour was the independent variable and coronary heart disease was the dependent variable.

Information overload A state that occurs when the individual is overwhelmed by incoming stimuli. It may occur when an anxious patient is overloaded with too much information at one time.

Institutionalisation A state that occurs when an individual is positively reinforced for being dependent upon the institution where he or she works or is a patient. The effect is insidious and is common in long-stay settings. It may affect both patients and staff.

Insulin A hormone secreted by the pancreas that regulates blood sugar or blood glucose. May be administered by injection for control of insulin-dependent diabetes.

Intellectualisation A mental defence mechanism that involves distancing oneself from patients emotionally and personally by viewing their condition as an intellectual problem.

Internal (self) standards The beliefs, values and attitudes that individuals acquire through experience. They are assumed to provide internal benchmarks that regulate the individual's behaviour.

Internal (person) variables A term used to describe any aspect of the self, such as an individual's traits, that can be used to explain behaviour.

Inter-personal A term meaning something shared between two or more individuals.

Intra-personal A term meaning within the individual, for example the private feeling of shame.

Large pain fibres A delta fibres that carry information about benign stimulation, such as itching. They have the hypothesised effect of closing the pain gate.

Law of effect Thorndike's theory or law which states that behaviour is modified by its consequences.

Lay-referral system The first source of information normally used when an individual is concerned about unusual symptoms. May be a friend, spouse, relative, work colleague, etc.

Learned helplessness A state that occurs when individuals perceive that they have no control over events.

Lesions A breakdown of tissue caused by disease, surgery or trauma.

Lifetime prevalence An estimate of the likelihood of a given disease or disorder occurring within an individual's lifetime.

Locus of control An important part of an individual's belief system that determines whether he or she believes that they have a great deal of personal control over events (internal locus of control) or that life is a series of uncontrollable, external events (external locus of control).

Longitudinal study A research methodology that involves following subjects or participants over a period of time, usually months or years. It is often used to chart developmental change.

Lumpectomy A surgical procedure for removing tumours from the breast. It is the least invasive procedure and involves removing the lump through a small incision in the areola of the nipple or under the flap of the breast.

Mental defence mechanisms Coping responses that lessen threats to the individual's self-concept. They are generally regarded as automatic or unconscious in that the individual is often unaware that they are being used.

Meylinisation The process wherein fatty sheaths are laid around fibres connecting neurones. Without their insulating properties, neurones cannot function properly.

Misattribution A term used when symptoms of illness are wrongly attributed to some other cause, such as age.

Morbidity A term used to describe a patient's physical prognosis or outlook following major illness or surgery.

Morphine A powerful, synthetic narcotic and analgesic, which occupies the receptor sites of naturally occurring opioids. Its side effects include respiratory depression and dependency.

Mortality A term used to describe the risk of death following, for example, major illness or surgery.

Mourning Culturally determined rituals that follow the death of an individual, for example the funeral, wearing mourning clothes, etc.

Multi-factorial A term often used in connection with diseases such as cancer that have multiple, rather than single, causes.

Multi-variate statistics A term used to describe statistical techniques that can be used to explore complex interactions between a large number of variables simultaneously.

Myocardial infarction An acute, life-threatening condition caused by sudden blocking of one or more of the coronary arteries resulting in tissue necrosis.

Natural killer cells A group of immune response cells that recognise tumours and lyse (break down) their cell membrane.

Nephritis Inflammation of the kidney.

Neuralgia An intermittent and idiosyncratic form of chronic pain.

Neural pathways Term used to describe the functional connections that link neurones and different regions of the brain.

Norepinephrine A 'stress hormone' secreted by the adrenal medulla. It raises heart rate and blood pressure and is also known by its proprietary name 'noradrenaline'. Its effects are similar to those of epinephrine.

Normative population A group, or population, of people used in a study in order to ascertain the normal (i.e. non-clinical or patho-logical) response to certain events or conditions.

Novel events A term used to describe events previously not experi-enced. They are often viewed as threatening because of the unknown challenges they may bring.

Nystagmus Rapid involuntary twitching of the eyeball.

Objective A measure or view that has been rationally or scientifically defined. It is assumed to be devoid of emotive content that might cause undue bias.

Oncology A term referring to the study and treatment of cancer.

Organic Meaning physical or biological in nature or origin.

Organisational variables A term used to describe organisational systems that increase compliance with health advice, such as primary nursing.

Pain behaviours Learned behaviours that include grimacing, attention-seeking and limping. Others' responses may positively reinforce such behaviours.

Parkinson's disease A chronic, degenerative disorder caused by a lack of dopamine in the brain controlling motor functions. Onset typically occurs later in life and it eventually affects cognitive as well as motor functioning.

Pattern theory of pain A pain theory that states that a single class of sensory receptors respond equally to pain, heat and touch stimuli.

Perceived control The individual's perception of how much control they have over certain events.

Perceived vulnerability A measure of how vulnerable or susceptible an individual feels with regard to a specific disease or condition.

Perception A term used to describe how the individual views or perceives the world. The assumption is that no two individuals perceive the world in exactly the same way.

Perioperative A term used to describe the period of time occurring immediately or shortly after surgery.

Personal coping style An individual's unique way(s) of dealing with stress.

Pessimism and fatalism A personality disposition associated with increased morbidity and mortality in patients with serious illness.

Phantom limb A phenomenon where the patient experiences sensations such as itching and (often intense) pain at the site of the amputated limb.

Phobia An intense, irrational fear of some object, person or thing.

Phylogenetic A term meaning 'across species'. For example, the brain stem is a phylogenetically ancient part of the brain found in all species of mammal.

Poliomyelitis A contagious viral disease that attacks the central nervous system causing temporary or permanent paralysis and weakness.

Positive reinforcement Anything or anyone that makes the recurrence of a behaviour or behaviours more likely.

Post traumatic stress disorder A chronic stress response that is characterised by emotional disturbance, intrusive thoughts and feelings of guilt.

Pre-conscious A term referring to thoughts, feelings and motives that are buried in the sub-conscious. They are regarded as having an automatic effect on behaviour, meaning that the individual is unaware of their operation. However, unlike *unconscious* thoughts and feelings, they are accessible to the individual through personal reflection.

Primacy-recency effect A psychological term used to describe the finding that people tend to remember the beginning and end of a chunk of information best, whilst tending to forget that which is placed in the middle.

Primary appraisal An initial judgement about whether or not a novel event poses a threat to well-being.

Private self-consciousness A psychological construct based on the premise that individuals high in PVSC are more introspective, i.e. aware of their thoughts, physical feelings and emotions.

Prospective study A study where baseline measurements of the experimental variables are taken at the start of a study.

Psychodynamic conflict A term used to describe conflict that arises when deep-seated desires conflict with that which is socially or personally acceptable.

Psychogenic A biological event, such as pain, that occurs in the absence of an obvious physical cause. Absence of a cause should not be used to infer that the symptoms do not exist.

Psychological construct A construct is an abstract concept that cannot be shown directly to exist. Examples are love, the self-concept and physical concepts like anti-matter. Their existence is inferred through other means, such as their effect on behaviour or other forms of matter.

Psychological event A term used to describe any event that has significant psychological consequences for the individual.

Psychosis A state where the individual loses contact with reality. It is characterised by a state of disorganisation, with auditory and (rarely) visual hallucinations, an inability to organise one's thoughts coherently and marked affective disturbance.

Public self-consciousness A psychological construct based on the premise that individuals high in PUBSC are overly concerned with their public image and others' reactions towards them.

Radical mastectomy A surgical procedure involving total removal of breast tissue and often the associated lymphatic tissue (i.e. the axillary nodes under the arm).

Reactive depression Depression that occurs as a reaction to events that typically involve loss. Also known as exogenous depression.

Recovery The final stage of Parkes' bereavement model.

Resilience A personality trait much like self-efficacy and hardiness, but it is assumed to have a strong biological basis.

Retrospective study An experimental study where the investigators try to ascertain the effect of an independent variable(s) on a dependent variable after the event has occurred.

Rumination A habitual tendency to engage in negative thinking (quite often regarding the self). It is commonly a feature of clinical depression.

Schizophrenia A disorder that is characterised by acute episodes wherein the individual becomes psychotic, has difficulty thinking logically and rationally and which is often accompanied by auditory hallucinations. A second type, 'negative schizophrenia', is less florid and is typified by loss of motivation and cognitive ability, and emotional flatness. Contrary to popular belief, it is not a 'split mind' syndrome.

Secondary appraisal A judgement occurring after a primary threat appraisal, that gauges whether or not the threat can be successfully dealt with.

Secondary gains A term used to describe a form of reinforcement that is derived from a state or condition that is normally regarded as aversive. Such gains may make the patient unwilling to get well and resume a normal life.

Self-concept The individual's sense of personal identity that includes body image, their beliefs, attitudes and values.

Self-consciousness An aversive experience that occurs in public situations as a consequence of fear of negative evaluation. It is characterised by feelings of anxiety, shyness and embarrassment.

Self-efficacy A personality trait or disposition that is characterised by a belief in one's ability to cope effectively with life events.

Self-esteem The affective component of the self. It is a feeling of self-worth that can be positive or negative.

Self-focused attention A term used to describe attentional processes fixed on some public or private aspect of the self.

Self-handicapping A mental defence mechanism wherein the individual creates conditions where failure is inevitable. In doing so, the conditions, rather than the self, can be blamed for the failure.

Self-monitoring A psychological construct that assumes individual differences in the extent to which people monitor and adjust their public image or behaviour.

Self-schema A psychological construct that contains information about aspects of self derived from past experience. Self-schemas are believed to affect the way in which we interpret and perceive information relevant to the self.

Self-serving bias An unconscious or automatic defence mechanism that leads individuals to attribute successes to internal factors and failures to external factors.

Sensory self-awareness A form of self-awareness that is limited to the sensory domain.

Shame A private, enduring and aversive experience that occurs as a consequence of some serious transgression of personal or cultural moral codes.

Sick role A state that occurs when a patient adopts the role of the invalid or patient and stops trying to achieve autonomy.

Significant others A term often used to describe people that are particularly influential in shaping behaviour, for example the parents, siblings and peers in the child's case.

Small diameter pain fibres A delta and C fibres that respond to sharp, localised pain and dull, diffuse pain respectively. Messages from these fibres are hypothesised to open the pain gate.

Social anxiety A class of anxiety evoked by the belief that the public image one wishes to present is likely to fail.

Social learning theory An influential theory that posits that significant others shape personality and behaviour during early childhood.

Social phobias A class of phobia that is characterised by a fear of public activities, such as eating, public speaking, etc.

Social referencing A form of learning wherein the infant observes the mother's non-verbal language as a means of ascertaining the safety, or otherwise, of the situation.

Somatic From the Greek word 'soma' meaning body. It is used to refer to the human body or the main part of individual cells.

Specificity theory of pain A pain theory stating that the brain has a specific centre dedicated to pain perception.

Stage models of loss Models of loss that describe stereotypical patterns of response that occur in relation to death and dying.

Stress A psychological construct that comprises a stressor, such as an aversive life event and stress response, which has a physical, emotional and behavioural component.

Subjective A measure or view that is personal and which is not deemed to have been rationally or scientifically defined. It is assumed that any emotive content might cause undue bias.

Subjective attitude A term used to describe attitudes held by others, particularly those who may influence a patient's health behaviour. Sometimes referred to as 'normative attitudes'.

Surgical resection Surgical removal of any part of the body or diseased tissue.

Systematic desensitisation A therapy for phobias that pairs a neutral stimulus with the aversive stimulus or stimuli responsible for the phobic reaction. Works on the premise that one cannot be relaxed and anxious simultaneously.

T cell An immune response cell that destroys the pathogen by phagocytosis (consuming the cell). The term is also used to describe the transmission cells hypothesised in the gate theory of pain.

Third factor variables A term used to describe any variable, other than the independent variable(s), that might affect the dependent variable in an experimental study.

Trait A unit of personality that represents an enduring and stable characteristic of an individual's behaviour.

Type A behaviour An identifiable pattern of habitual behaviour that is believed to increase the risk of coronary heart disease.

Variable Something that varies in relation to something else. For example, sleep is a variable that is typically affected by the variable caffeine.

Venipuncture Puncture of a vein with a needle or cannula.

Vicarious reinforcement A type of learning that occurs following mere observation of someone or something performing a particular behaviour.

References

Abramson, I. Y., Seligman, M. E. and Teasdale, E. J. (1978). Learned helplessness in humans: Critique and reformulation. *Journal of Abnormal Psychology*. 87, 49–74.

Agras, S. (1969). The epidemiology of common fears and phobias. *Comprehensive Psychiatry*. 10, 151–156.

Ainsworth, M. D. S. (1982). Attachment: Retrospect and prospect. In Parkes, C. M. and Stevenson-Hinde, L. (Eds). *The Place of Attachment in Human Behaviour*. London: Tavistock.

Ainsworth, M. D. S., Blehar M. C. and Wall, S. (1978). *Patterns of Attachment: A Psychological Study of the strange situation*. Hillsdale NJ: Erlbaum.

Ajzen, I. (1985). From interventions to action: A theory of planned behaviour. In Kuhl, J. and Beckman, J. (Eds). *Action Control*. New York: Springer.

Ajzen, I. and Fishbein, M. (1980). *Understanding Attitudes and Predicting Social Behaviour*. Englewood Cliffs, NJ: Prentice Hall.

Alexander, F. (1950). *Psychosomatic Medicine*. New York: Norton.

Alloy, L. B. and Abramson, L. Y. (1979). Judgement contingency in depressed and non-depressed students: Sadder but wiser? *Journal of Experimental Psychology: General*. 108, 441–485.

Alter, C. L., Pelcovitz, P., Axelrod, B. and Goldenberg, B. (1996). Identification of post traumatic stress disorder in cancer survivors. *Psychosomatics*. 37, 2: 137–143.

Anderson, K. O., Dowds, B. N., Pelletz, R.E., Edwards, W. T. and Peeters-Asdourian, C. (1995). Development and initial validation of a scale to measure self-efficacy beliefs in patients with chronic pain. *Pain*. 63, 77–84.

Antonovosky, A. and Hartman, H. (1974). Delay in detection of cancer: A review. *Health Education Monographs*. 2, 98–125.

Argyle, M. (1983). *The Psychology of Interpersonal Behaviour*. London: Pelican.

REFERENCES

Asendorpf, J. (1990). The expression of shyness and embarrassment. In Crozier, R. W. (Ed). *Shyness and Embarrassment: Perspectives from social psychology.* Cambridge: Cambridge University Press.

Atkinson, R. L., Atkinson, R. C., Smith, E. E. and Bem, D. J. (1993). *Introduction to Psychology.* 11th ed. Fort Worth: Harcourt, Brace Jovanovich.

Bakal, D. A. (1979). *Psychology and Medicine: Psychological dimensions of health and illness.* New York: Springer.

Bandura, A. (1977). Self-efficacy: Towards a unifying theory of behavioural change. *Psychological Review.* 84, 191–215.

Bandura, A. (1986). *Social Foundations of Thought and Action: A social cognitive model.* Englewood Cliffs, NJ: Prentice Hall.

Bandura, A., O'Leary, A., Taylor, C. B., Ganthies, J. and Gossard, G. (1987). Perceived self-efficacy and pain control: opioid and non-opioid mechanisms. *Journal of Personality and Social Psychology.* 53, 563–571.

Bartrop, R. W., Luckhurst, E. and Lazarus, L. (1977). Depressed lymphocyte function after bereavement. *Lancet.* 1, 834–836.

Bates, E., O'Connol, B. and Shore, C. (1987). Language and communication in infancy. In Osefsky, J. D. (Ed). *Handbook of Infant Development.* 2nd ed. New York: Wiley Interscience.

Beck, A. T. (1976). *Cognitive Therapy and Emotional Disorders.* New York: International Universities Press.

Beck, A. T. (1987). Cognitive models of depression. *Journal of Cognitive Psychotherapy: An International Quarterly.* 1, 5–37.

Beck, A. T. and Emery, G. E. (1985). *Anxiety Disorders and Phobias: A cognitive perspective.* New York: Basic Books.

Becker, M. H. and Rosenstock, I. M. (1984). Compliance with medical advice. In Steptoe, A. and Mathews, A. (Eds). *Health Care and Human Behaviour.* London: Academic Press.

Bee, H. (1997). *The Developing Child.* 8th ed. New York: HarperCollins.

Beecher, H. K. (1956). Relationship of significance of wound to pain experienced. *Journal of American Medical Association.* 161, 1609–1613.

Bem, D. J. (1972). Self-perception theory. In Berkowitz, L. (Ed). *Advances in Experimental Psychology (Vol. 6).* New York: Academic Press.

Benjamin, P. (1978). Psychological problems following recovery from acute life-threatening illness. *American Journal of Orthopsychiatry.* 48, 284–290.

Benner, P. (1984). *From novice to expert: Excellence and power in clinical practice.* Menlo Park: Addison-Wesley.

Benner, P. A., Tanner, C. A., and Chelsa, C. A. (1987). *Expertise in Nursing Practice.* New York: Springer Publishing Co.

Bennet, P. and Murphy. S. (1997). *Psychology and Health Promotion.* Buckingham: Open University Press.

Berkman, L. F. (1995). The role of social relations in health promotion. *Psychosomatic Medicine.* 57, 245–254.

Berkowitz, A. (1993). *Aggression: Its causes, consequences and control.* New York: McGraw Hill.

Bernstein, I. L. (1978). Learned taste aversion in children receiving chemotherapy. *Science.* 200, 1302–1303.

Bibbace, R. and Walsh, M. E. (1980). Development of children's concepts of illness. *Paediatrics.* 66, 912–917.

Bilton, T., Bonnett, K., Jones, P. *et al.* (1987). *Introductory Sociology.* 2nd ed. Basingstoke: Macmillan Press.

Birren, J. E. and Schaie, K. W. (1985). *Handbook of Ageing*. 2nd ed. San Diego: Academic Press.

Birren, J. E. and Schaie, K. W. (1990). *Handbook of Ageing*. 3rd ed. San Diego: Academic Press.

Bloom, F. E., Lazerson, A. and Hoftader, L. (1985). *Brain, Mind and Behaviour*. New York: Freeman.

Boston, K., Pearce, I. B. and Richardson, P. H. (1990). The pain cognitions questionnaire. *Journal of Psychosomatic Research*. 34, 103–109.

Botwinick, J. (1977). *Aging and Human Behaviour*. New York: Springer.

Bowlby, J. (1969). *Attachment and Loss. Vol 1. Attachment*. New York: Basic Books.

Bowlby, J. (1975). *Attachment and Loss. Vol 2. Separation, anxiety and anger*. New York: Basic Books.

Bowlby, J. (1980). *Attachment and Loss. Vol 3. Loss, sadness and depression*. New York: Basic Books.

Bowling, A. (1991). *Measuring Health. A Review of Quality of Life Measurement Scales*. Buckingham: Open University Press.

Bradbury, E, (1993). Psychological approaches to children with disfigurement. *ACCP Review and Newsletter*. 15, vol. 1.

Brewin. C. R. (1988). *Cognitive Foundations of Clinical Psychology*. Hove: Erlbaum.

Broadbent, D. E. (1958). *Perception and Communication*. London: Pergamon.

Bromley, D. B. (1988). *Human Ageing*. Harmondsworth: Penguin.

Brown, G. W. (1982). Early social loss and depression. In Parkes, C. M. and Stevenson-Hinde, L. (Eds). *The Place of Attachment in Human Behaviour*. London: Tavistock.

Brown, G. W. and Harris, T. O. (1978). *Social Origins of Depression*. London; Tavistock.

Bunney, W. E., Goodwin, F. K. and Murphy, D. L. (1970) The switch process from depression to mania: Relationship to drugs that alter brain amines. *Lancet*. 1, 1022.

Buss, A. (1980). *Self-consciousness and Social Anxiety*. New York: W. H. Freeman; Cambridge: Cambridge University Press.

Buss, A. and Plomin, R. (1984). *Temperament: Early developing personality traits*. Hillsdale, NJ: Erlbaum.

Butler, R. W., Rizzi, L. P. and Handwerger, B. A. (1996). Cancer in children and post-traumatic stress disorder. *Journal of Paediatric Psychology*. 21 (4), 499–504.

Cannon, W. B. (1927). As cited in Atkinson, R. L., Atkinson, R. C., Smith, E. E. and Bem, D. J. (1993). *Introduction to Psychology*. 11th ed. Fort Worth: Harcourt, Brace Jovanovich.

Caplan, G. (1964). *Principles of Preventative Psychiatry*. New York: Basic Books.

Carr, A. T. (1981). Dying and bereavement. In Griffiths, D. (Ed). *Psychology and Medicine*. London: British Psychological Society/Macmillan.

Carr, A. T. (1982). Dying and bereavement. Chapter 17. In Hall, J. (Ed). *Psychology for Nurses and Health Visitors*. London: British Psychological Society/Macmillan Press.

Castalfranchi, C. and Poggi, I. (1990). Blushing as a discourse: was Darwin wrong? In Crozier, R. W. (Ed). *Shyness and Embarrassment: Perspectives from social psychology*. Cambridge: Cambridge University Press.

Chapman, C. R. and Bronica, J. J. (1985). *Chronic Pain*. Kalamazoo, MI: Upjohn.

Chapman, S. L. and Brena, S. F. (1985). Pain and society. *Annals of Behavioural Medicine*. 7 (3), 21–24.

Cheek, J. M. and Buss, A. H. (1981) Shyness and sociability. *Journal of Personality and Social Psychology*. 41 (2), 330–339.

Cheek, J. and Melchoir, L. A. (1990). Shyness, self-esteem and self-consciousness. In Leitenberg, L. A. (Ed). *Handbook of Evaluation Anxiety*. New York: Plenum Press.

Clausen, J. and Radke Yarrow, M. (1985). The impact of mental illness on the family. *Journal of Social Issues*. 11, 1–10.

Cohen, F. and Lazarus, R. S. (1983). Coping and adaptation in health and illness. In Mechanic, D. (Ed). *Handbook of Health Care and the Health Professions*. New York: Free Press.

Cohen, J. B. and Reed, D. (1984). The type A behaviour and coronary heart disease risk amongst Japanese men in Hawaii. *Journal of Behavioural Medicine*. 8, 343–352.

Cohen, S. and Wills, T. A. (1985). Stress, social support and the buffering hypothesis. *Psychological Bulletin*. 98, 310–357.

Cohn, D. A. (1990). Child–mother attachment of six-year-olds and social competence at school. *Child Development*. 61, 151–162.

Collier, J. (1997). Developing a generic quality of life measure. *Health Psychology Update*. BPS Special Group in Health Psychology. Issue 28, June.

Conduit, E. H. (1992). If A-B does not predict heart disease why bother with it? *British Journal of Medical Psychology*. 65 (3), 289–296.

Conway, M. A., Gardiner, J. M., Anderson, S. J. and Cohen, N. (in press). Memory awareness and learning. *Journal of Exprimental Psychology*.

Cooley, C.H. (1902). As cited in Staub, E. (1980). *Personality: Basic concepts and current research*. Engelwood Cliffs, NJ: Prentice Hall.

Coons, H. L., Leventhal, H., Nerenz, D. R. (1990). Anticipatory nausea and emotional distress in patients receiving Cisplastic-based chemotherapy. *Oncology Forum*.

Coopersmith, S. (1967). *The Antecedents of Self-esteem*. San Francisco: Freeman.

Cox, J. and Holden, J. (1994). *Perinatal Psychiatry: Use and misuse of the Edinburgh Post Natal Depression Scale*. Royal College of Psychiatrists. London: Gaskell.

Cox, T. (1978). *Stress*. Baltimore: University Park Press.

Cromer, R. J. (1996). *Fundamentals of Abnormal Psychology*. New York: W. H. Freeman.

Crozier, R. W. (1982). Explanations of social shyness. *Current Psychological Reviews*. 2, 47–60.

Davidson, G. C. and Neale, J. M. (1982). *Abnormal Psychology*. 3rd ed. New York: John Wiley.

Davidson, G. C. and Neale, J. M. (1994). *Abnormal Psychology*. 6th ed. New York: John Wiley.

Davidson, J. R. T. and Foa, E. B. F. (1993). *Post Partum Psychosis: Beyond DSM IV*. Washington: Psychiatric Press.

Davies, A. D. M. (1996). In Woods, T. (Ed). *Handbook of Clinical Psychology of Ageing*. Chichester: John Wiley.

Davis, M. S. (1966). Variations in patient compliance with doctor's advice. *American Journal of Public Health*. 58, 274–288.

Davis, M. S. (1968). Variations in patients' compliance with doctors' advice. *American Journal of Public Health* 58, 274–288.

Davitz. J. R. (1952). The effect of precision training on postfrustration behaviour. *Journal of Abnormal and Social Psychology*. 47, 309–315.

Deaux, K. (1984). From individual differences to social categories: An analysis of a decade's research on gender. *American Psychologist*. 39 (2), 105–115.

Devellis, R. F., Devellis, B. M., Wallston, B. S. and Wallston, K. A. (1980). Epilepsy and learned helplessness. *Basic and Applied Social Psychology*. 1, 243–253.

Diagnostic and Statistical Manual of Mental Disorders. (DSM IV). (1994). Washington: American Psychiatric Association.

Dickstein, S. and Park, R. D. (1988). Social referencing in infancy. *Child Development*. 59, 506–511.

DiMatteo, M. D. and DiNichola, D. D. (1982). *Achieving Patient Compliance: The psychology of the medical practitioner's role*. New York: Pergamon Press.

Dolgin, M. J., Katz, E. R., McGinty, K. and Seigel, S. E. (1986). Anticipatory nausea and vomiting in paediatric cancer patients. Unpublished manuscript. As cited in Johnston, M. and Wallace, L. (1990). (Eds). *Stress and Medical Procedures*. Oxford: Oxford University Press.

Dollard, J., Doob, L., Miller, N. E., *et al.* (1939). *Frustration and Aggression*. New Haven: Yale University Press.

Dougher, M. J., Gouldstein, D. and Leight, K. A. (1987). Induced anxiety and pain. *Journal of Anxiety Disorders*. 1, 259–264.

Douglas, J. E. and Byron, M. (1996). Interview data on severe eating difficulties in young children. *Archives of Diseases in Childhood*. 75, 304–308.

Draper, P. (1997). *Nursing Perspectives on Quality of Life*. London: Routledge.

Dreyfus, H. L. and Dreyfus, S. E. (1996). The relationship of theory and practice in the acquisition of skill. In Benner, P. A., Tanner, C. A. and Chelsa, C. A. (1996). *Expertise in Nursing Practice: Caring, clinical judgement and ethics*. New York: Springer.

Dubner, R. and Ruda, M. A. (1992). Activity dependent neuronal plasticity following tissue injury and inflammation. *Trends in Neurosciences*. 15, 96–103.

Duval, S. and Wicklund, R. (1972). *A Theory of Objective Self-awareness*. New York: Academic Press.

Edelman, R. J. (1981). Embarrassment: The state of research. *Current Psychological Reviews*. 1, 125–138.

Eiser, C. (1994). What do children mean by quality of life? *Health Psychology Update*. BPS Special Group in Health Psychology. Issue 16, June.

Ellis, A. (1962). *Reason and Emotion in Psychotherapy*. New York: Lyle-Stuart.

Ellis, A. (1977). The basic clinical theory of rationale-emotive therapy. In Ellis, A. and Grieger, R. (Eds). *Handbook of Rational Emotive Therapy*. New York: Springer.

Emde, R. N. (1985). In Tuma, A. H. and Maser, J. D. (Eds). *Anxiety and Anxiety Disorders*. Hillsdale, NJ: Erlbaum.

Erikson, E.H. (1950). *Childhood and Society*. New York: Norton.

Fallon, A. (1990). In Cash, T. F. and Pruzinsky, T. (Eds). *Body Image: Development deviance and change*. New York: Guilford Press.

Farber, B. A. (1989). Psychological mindedness: Can there be too much of a good thing? *Psychotherapy* 26 (2), 210–217.

Fawzy, F. I., Fawzy, N. W. and Hyun, C. S. (1993). Malignant melanoma: Effects of an early structured intervention, coping and affective state on recurrence and survival 6 years later. *Archives of General Psychiatry*. 50, 681–689.

Feldman, R. S. (1995). *Social Psychology*. Englewood Cliffs, NJ: Prentice Hall.

Fellner, C. H. and Marshall, J. R. (1970). Kidney donors. In Macauley, J. and Berkowitz, L. (Eds). *Altruism and Helping Behaviour*. New York: Academic Press.

Fenigstein, A. (1979). Self-consciousness, self-attention and social interaction. *Journal of Personality and Social Psychology*. 37, 75–86.

Fenigstein, A., Scheier, M. F. and Buss, A. H. (1975). Public and private self-consciousness: Assessment and theory. *Journal of Consulting and Clinical Psychology*. 43 (4), 522–527.

Festinger. L. (1954). A theory of social comparative processes. *Human Relations*. 7 (3), 117–140.

Field, T. (1989). Maternal depression effects on infant interaction and attachment behaviour. In Ciccehti, D. (Ed). *The Emergence of a Discipline. Vol 1*. Hillsdale, NJ: Erlbaum.

Field, T., Healy, B., Goldstein, S. and Guthertz, M. (1990). Behaviour-state matching and synchrony in mother–infant interactions of nondepressed versus depressed dyads. *Developmental Psychology*. 26, 7–14.

Fields, H. L. and Levine, J. D. (1984). Placebo in analgesia: A role for endorphins? *Trends in Neuroscience*. 7, 271–273.

Firth, H. and Rapley. M. (1990). *From Acquaintance to Friendship: Issues for people with learning disabilities*. Kidderminster: BMH Publications.

Fisher, S. (1973) *Body Consciousness*. London: Open Forum.

Fiske, S. T. and Taylor, S. E. (1984). *Social Cognition*. New York: London House.

Flor, H., Kerns, R. D. and Turk, D. C. (1987). The role of spouse reinforcement, perceived pain and activity levels of chronic pain patients. *Journal of Psychosomatic Research*. 31, 251–259.

Folks, D. G., Freeman, A. M., Sokol, R. S. and Thurstin, A. H. (1988). Denial: Prediction of outcome following coronary bypass surgery. *International Journal of Psychiatry in Medicine*. 18 (1), 55–66.

Fordyce, W. E. (1976). *Behavioural Methods in Chronic Pain and Illness*. St Louis: Mosby.

Fordyce, W. E. and Steger, J. C. (1979). Behavioural management of chronic pain. In Pomerleau, O. F. and Brady. J. P. (Eds). *Behavioural Medicine: Theory and practice*. Baltimore: Williams and Wilkins.

Fraiberg, S. (1975). The development of human attachments in infants blind from birth. *Merril-Palmer Quarterly*. 21, 315–334.

Friedman, M. and Rosenman, R. H. (1960). Western Collaborative Group Study. As cited in Kaplan, R. M., Sallis, J. F. and Patterson, T. L. (1993). *Health and Human Behaviour*. New York: McGraw-Hill.

Friedman, M. and Rosenman, R. H. (1974). *Type A Behaviour and Your Heart*. New York: Knopf.

Freud, S. (1901/1960). *Psychopathology of Everyday Life*. (Standard ed.) (*Vol. 6*). London: Hogarth Press.

Garfinkel, P. E. and Garner, M. G. (1982). *Anorexia Nervosa: A multidimensional perspective*. Montreal: Bruner/Mazel Publishers.

Garrity, T. and Garrity, M. (1985). Cited in Pitts, M. and Phillips, K. (Eds) *The Psychology of Health*. London: Routledge.

Garmezy, N. (1983). Stressors in childhood. In Garmezy, N. and Rutter, M. (Eds). *Stress, Coping and Development in Children*. New York: McGraw-Hill.

Gatchel, R. J., Baum, A. and Krantz, D. S. (1989). *An Introduction to Health Psychology*. London: McGraw-Hill.

Geersten, H. R., Gray, R.M. and Ward, J. R. Patient non-compliance within the context of seeking medical care for arthritis. *Journal of Chronic Diseases*. 26, 689–698.

Gergen, K. J. (1971). *The Concept of Self*. New York: Holt, Reinhart and Winston.

Gibbons, F. X. (1990). The impact of focus of attention and affect on social behaviour. In Crozier, R. W. (Ed). *Shyness and Embarrassment: Perspectives from social psychology*. Cambridge: Cambridge University Press.

Gill, K. M., Keefe, F. J., Sampson, H. A., McCaskil, C. C. *et al.* (1988). Direct observation of scratching behaviour in children with atopic dermatitis. *Behaviour Therapy*. 19, 213–227.

Goffman, E. (1959). *The Presentation of Self in Everyday Life*. New York: Doubleday-Anchor Books.

Goffman, E. (1961). *Asylums: Essays on the social situations of mental patients*. New York: Doubleday-Anchor Books.

Glass, D. C. (1977). *Behaviour Patterns, Stress and Coronary Heart Disease*. Hillsdale, NJ: Elrbaum.

Goldbeck-Wood, S. (1996). PTSD and childbirth. *British Medical Journal*. 313, 7060–7074.

Grace, W. J. and Graham, D. T. (1952). The relationship of specific attitudes and emotions to certain bodily diseases. *Psychosomatic Medicine*. 29, 52–71.

Greer, S. and Morris, T. (1975). Psychological attributes of women who develop breast cancer: A controlled study. *Journal of Psychosomatic Research*. 19, 147–153.

Grosarth-Maticek, R., Kanariz, D. T., Schmidt, P. *et al.* (1982a). Psychosomatic processes in the development of cancerogenesis. *Psychotherapy Psychosomatics*. 38, 284–302.

Grosarth-Maticek, R., Seigrist, J. and Vetter, H. (1982b). Interpersonal repression as a predictor of cancer. *Social Science and Medicine*. 16, 493–498.

Guyton, A. C. (1985). *Anatomy and Physiology*. Philadelphia: Saunders.

Hamilton, S. (1996). In Woods, T. (Ed). *Handbook of Clinical Psychology of Ageing*. Chichester: John Wiley.

Harré, R. (1990). In Crozier, R. W. (Ed). *Shyness and Embarrassment: Perspectives from social psychology*. Cambridge: Cambridge University Press.

Harter, S. (1983). Developmental perspectives on the self-system. In P. H. Mussen (Ed.). *Handbook of Child Psychology*. 4th ed. New York: John Wiley.

Harter, S. (1985). Competence as a dimension of self-evaluation: Towards a comprehensive model of self-worth. In Leahy, R. L. (Ed). *The development of the Self*. Orlando, FL: Academic Press.

Harter, S. (1988a). The determinations and mediations of global self-worth in children. In Eisenberg, N. (Ed). *Contemporary Topics in Developmental Psychology*. New York: Wiley-Interscience.

Harter, S. (1988b). Developmental processes in the construction of the self. In Yankey, T. D. and Johnson, J. E. (Eds). *Integrative Processes and Socialism: Early to middle childhood*. New York: John Wiley.

Hastrup, K. (1995). In Cohen, A. P. and Rapport, N. (Eds). *Questions of Consciousness*. Routledge: London.

Hastrup, S. (1993). Peer relations. In Mussen, P. H. (Ed) *Handbook of Child Psychology*. 4th ed. New York: John Wiley.

Haynes, S., Feinleib, M. and Kannel (1980). The relationship of psychosocial factors to coronary heart disease in the Framingham Study. III: Eight year incidence of CHD. *American Journal of Epidemiology.* 107, 37–58.

Hayslip, B. and Panek, P. E. (1993). *Adult Development and Ageing.* New York: HarperCollins.

Herbert, M. (1996). *ABC of Behavioural Methods.* Leicester: BPS Books.

Higgins, E. T. (1990) as cited in Crozier, R. W. (Ed). *Shyness and Embarrassment: Perspectives from social psychology.* Cambridge: Cambridge University Press.

Hilgard, E. R. and Hilgard, J. R. (1983). *Hypnosis and the Relief of Pain.* (rev. ed.) Los Altos, CA: Kaufmann.

Hobson, R. P. (1993). *Autism and the Development of the Mind.* Hove: Erlbaum.

Horn, J. L. and Cattel, R. B. (1966). Refinement and test of the theory of fluid and crystallised general intelligence. *Journal of Educational Psychology.* 57, 253–270.

Horn, J. L. and Donaldson, G. (1976). On the myth of intellectual decline in adulthood. *American Psychologist.* 31, 701–709.

Horn, S. and Munafó, M. (1997). *Pain: Theory research and intervention.* Buckingham: Open University Press.

Horowitz, M. (1975). Intensive and repetitive thoughts after experimental stress. *Archives of General Psychiatry.* 32, 1457–1463.

Howard, R. W. (1987). *Concepts and Schemata: An introduction.* Cassell Education.

Hughes, J., Smith, T. W. and Kosterlitz, H. W. (1975). Identification of two related pentapeptides from the brain with opioid activity. *Journal of Gerontology.* 40, 268–274.

Hyland, M. and Donaldson, M. (1989). *Psychological Care in Nursing Practice.* London: Scatari Press.

Ingram, R. E. (1970). Attentional specificity in depressive and generalised anxiety states. *Cognitive Therapy and Research.* 14 (1). 25–31.

Irwin, M., Daniels, M., Bloom, E. *et al.* (1987). Life events, depression symptoms and immune function. *American Journal of Psychiatry.* 144, 437–431.

Jacobsen, E. (1983). *Progressive Relaxation.* Urbana, IL: University of Chicago Press.

James, A. (1995). In Cohen, A. P. and Rapport, N. (Eds). *Questions of Consciousness.* Routledge: London.

Janis, I. L. (1958). *Psychological Stress: Psychoanalytic and behavioural studies of surgical patients.* London: Chapman.

Janis, I. L. and Mann, L. (1979). *Decision Making.* New York: Free Press.

Janz, N. K. and Becker, M. H. (1984). The health belief model: A decade later. *Health Education Quarterly.* 11 (1), 1–47.

Johal, S. (1995). Quality of life: an evaluation alternative for genetic services. *Health Psychology Update.* BPS Special Group in Health Psychology. Issue 20, June.

Johnston, M. and Wallace, L. (1990). *Stress and Medical Procedures.* Oxford: Oxford University Press.

Jones, E. E. and Pittman, T. S. (1982). Towards a theory of strategic self-presentation. In Suls, J. (Ed.). *Psychological Perspectives on the Self.* Hillsdale, NJ: Erlbaum.

Joseph, S., Williams, R. and Yule, W. (1997). *Understanding Post Traumatic Stress Disorder: A psychosocial perspective on PTSD and treatment.* Chichester: John Wiley.

Kagan, C. (1987). Teaching interpersonal skills. In Muller, D. (Ed). *Teaching Psychological Skills to Nurses.* Leicester: British Psychological Society.

Kagan, J. (1982). The emergence of the self. *Journal of Child Psychiatry and Psychology*. 23, 363–381.

Kahana, E. and Kahana, B. (1982). Environmental continuity, futurity and adaptation of the aged. In Rowles, G. and Ohta, K. (Eds). *Ageing and Milieu*. New York: Academic Press.

Kahneman, D. and Tversky, A. (1982). On the study of statistical intuitions. In Kahneman, D., Slovic, P. and Tversky, A. *Judgements under Uncertainty: Heuristics and biases*. Cambridge: Cambridge University Press.

Kaplan, R. M., Sallis, J. F. and Patterson, T. L. (1993). *Health and Human Behaviour*. New York: McGraw-Hill.

Karoly, P. (1985). *Measurement Strategies in Health Psychology*. New York: Wiley.

Keinen, G., Ben-Zur, H. and Carel, R. S. (1992). Looking for 'FIDO': Evaluating research on expressed anger in the pathogenesis of coronary heart disease. *Psychology and Health*. 7, 83–98.

Kelly, M. P. and May, D. (1982). Good and bad patients: A review of the literature and theoretical critique. *Journal of Advanced Nursing*. 7, 147–156.

Kendell-Tackett, K. A. and Kaufman-Kantor, G. (1993). *Postpartum Depression: A comprehensive approach for nurses*. London: Sage.

Kermis, M. (1984). *Psychology of Human Ageing: Theory research and practice*. Barton: Allyn and Bacon.

Kiecolt-Glaser, J. K. and Glaser, R. G. (1995). Psychoneuroimmunology and health consequences: Data and shared mechanisms. *Psychosomatic Medicine*. 57, 269–274.

Kiecolt-Glaser, J. K., Garner, W. and Speicher, C. E. (1984). Psychosocial modifiers of social stress in medical students. *Psychosomatic Medicine*. 46, 7–14.

Kimmel, D. C. (1990). *Adulthood and Ageing*. New York: HarperCollins.

Kobasa, S. C. (1979). Stressful life events, personality and health: An inquiry into hardiness. *Journal of Personality and Social Psychology*. 37, 1–11.

Kraft, T. (1993). A case of chemotherapy phobia: An integrative approach. *Contemporary-Hypnosis*. 10 (2), 105–111.

Kubler-Ross, E. (1969). *On Death and Dying*. London: Tavistock.

Lachman, M. E. (1968). Locus of contol in ageing research. *Psychology and Aging*. 1, 34–40.

Lancaster, J. L. (1984). *Adult Psychiatric Nursing*. New York: Medical Examination Publishing Co.

Lau, R. R. and Hartman, K. A. (1983). Common sense representations of illness. *Health Psychology*. 2, 167–185.

Lazarus, A. A. (1971). *Behaviour Therapy and Beyond*. New York: McGraw-Hill.

Lazarus, R. S. (1983). The costs and benefits of denial. In Brenitz, S. (Ed.). *In the Denial of Stress*. New York: International Press.

Lazarus, R. S. and Folkman, S. (1984). *Stress, Appraisal and Coping*. New York: Springer.

Lecky, P. (1969). As cited in Staub, E. (1980). *Personality: Basic concepts and current research*. Englewood Cliffs, NJ: Prentice Hall.

Lerner, M. J. (1975). The justice motive in social behaviour. *Journal of Social Issues*. 31, 3: 1–19.

Letemendia, M. (1985). An age old problem. *Nursing Times*. April, 24, 30–32.

Leventhal, H., Benyamini, Y. and Brownlea, S. *et al.* (1997). In Petrie, K. J. and Weinman, J. A. (Eds). *Perception of Health and Illness*. London: Harvard.

Levine, J., Warrenburg, S., Kerns, R., Delaney, R. *et al.* (1987). The role of denial in recovery from CHD. *Psychosomatic Medicine*. 49 (2), 109–117.

Lewinsohn, P. M. and Mischel, W. (1980). Social competence and depression: The role of illusory self-perceptions. *Journal of Abnormal Psychology*, 89 (2), 203–212.

Lewis, M. and Brooks-Gunn, J. (1979). *Social Cognition and Acquisition of Self*. New York: Plenum.

Ley, P. (1982). Satisfaction, compliance and communication. *British Journal of Social and Clinical Psychology*. 21, 241–254.

Ley, P. and Spelman, M. S. (1967). Communications in an out-patient setting. *British Journal of Social and Clinical Psychology*. 4, 114–116.

Luthe, W. and Schultz, J. H. (1969). *Autogenic Therapy*. New York: Grune and Stratton.

McCrae, R. R. and Costa, P. J. Jr (1987). Validation of the five-factor model of personality across instruments and observers. *Journal of Personality and Social Psychology*, 52, 81–90.

McKinnon, W., Weisse, C. S. and Reynolds, C. P. (1989). Chronic stress, leukocyte sub-populations and humoral response to latent viruses. *Health Psychology*. 8, 389–402.

Main, M. and Weston, D. R. (1982) Avoidance of the attachment figure in infancy. In Parkes, C. M. and Stevenson-Hinde, L. (Eds). *The Place of Attachment in Human Behaviour*. London: Tavistock.

Marcia, J. E. (1980). Identity in adolescence. In Adelson, J. (Ed). Handbook of Adolescent Psychology. New York: John Wiley.

Mark, J., Williams, G., Fraser, W., Watts, A. and Mathew, A. (1997). *Cognitive Psychology and Emotional Disorders*. 2nd ed. Chichester: John Wiley.

Marks, I. M. (1987). *Fears, Phobias and Rituals*. New York: Oxford University Press.

Marks, I. M. (1997). *Living with Fear: Understanding and coping with anxiety*. Maidenhead: McGraw Hill.

Markus, H. and Nurius, A. (1986). Possible selves. *American Psychologist*. 41 (9), 954–969.

Markus, H. and Sentis, K. (1982). The self in social information processing. In Suls, J. (Ed). *Psychological Perspectives on the Self*. Vol. 1. Hillsdale, NJ: Erlbaum.

Martin, G. and Pear, J. (1996). *Behaviour Modification: What it is and how to do it*. 5th ed. New Jersey: Prentice Hall.

Maslow, A. H. (1970). *Motivation and Personality* (2nd ed.). New York: Harper and Row.

Masters, J. C. and Smith, W. P. (1987). *Social Comparison, Social Justice and Relative Deprivation*. Hillsdale, NJ: Erlbaum.

Mathews, K. A. and Haynes, S. G. (1986). Type A behaviour pattern and coronary disease risk: Update and critical evaluation. *American Journal of Epidemiology*. 123, 923–960.

May, R. (1972). *Power and Innocence: A search for the sources of violence*. New York: Norton.

Mead, G. H. (1934). As cited in Staub, E. (1980). *Personality: Basic concepts and current research*. Englewood Cliffs, NJ: Prentice Hall.

Mead, N., Bower, P. and Gask, L. (1997). Emotional problems in primary care: What is the potential for increasing the role of the nurse? *Journal of Advanced Nursing*. 26 879–890.

Meichenbuam, D. (1977) *Cognitive Behaviour Modification*. New York: Plenum.

Meichenbaum, D. and Turk, D. C. (1986). *Facilitating Treatment Adherence*. New York: Plenum.

Melamed, B. G. and Siegel, L. J. (1985). Children's reactions to medical stressors. In Tumas, A. H. and Maser, J. D. (Eds). *Anxiety and Anxiety Disorders*. Hillsdale, NJ: Erlbaum.

Melzack, R. and Wall, P. D. (1965). Pain mechanisms: A new theory. *Science*. 150, 971–979.

Melzack, R. and Wall, P. D. (1982). *The Challenge of Pain*. New York: Basic Books.

Metalsky, G. I., Halberstadt, L. J. and Abramson, I. Y. (1987). Vulnerability and invulnerability to depressive mood reactions. *Journal of Personality and Social Psychology*. 52, 386–393.

Meyer, D., Leventhal, H. and Guttman, M. (1985). Common sense models of illness. *Health Psychology*. 2, 117–132.

Miller, N. E. (1941). The frustration-aggression hypothesis. *Psychological Review*. 48, 337–340.

Mischel, W. (1973). Towards a cognitive social learning re-conceptualisation of personality. *Psychological Review*. 80, 272–283.

Montemayor, R. and Eisen, M. (1977). The development of self-conceptions from childhood to adolescence. *Developmental Psychology*. 13, 314–319.

Moos, R. (1982). Coping with acute health crises. In Millon, T., Green, C. and Meagher, R. (Eds). (1982). *Handbook of Clinical Health Psychology*. New York: Plenum.

Mowrer, O. H. (1947). On the dual nature of learning – a reinterpretation of conditioning and problem solving. *Harvard Educational Review*. 17, 102–148.

Nichols, K. A. (1985). Psychological care for nurses, paramedical and medical staff: Essential developments for general hospitals. *British Journal of Medical Psychology*. 58, 241–248.

Niven, N. (1989). *Health Psychology: An introduction for nurses and health professionals*. Edinburgh: Churchill Livingstone.

Nowakowski, R. S. (1987). Basic concepts of CNS development. *Child Development*. 58, 568–595.

Parkes, C. M. (1972). *Bereavement: Studies of grief in adult life*. London: Tavistock.

Parkes, C. M. (1986). 3rd ed. *Bereavement: Studies of grief in adult life*. London: Tavistock.

Parkes, C. M. and Weiss, R. S. (1983). *Recovery from Bereavement*. New York: Basic Books.

Parsons, T. (1951). *The Social System*. Glencoe, IL: Free Press.

Pavlov, I. D. (1927). Conditioned Responses. New York: Oxford University Press.

Pelcovitz, C., Goldenberg, B. and Caplan, S. (1996). Post traumatic stress disorder in mothers of paediatric cancer survivors. *Psychosomatics*. 37 (2), 116–126.

Piaget, J. (1954). *The Construction of Reality in the Child*. New York: Basic Books.

Pitts, M. (1991). The experience of treatment. In Pitts, M. and Phillips, K. (Eds) *The Psychology of Health*. London: Routledge.

Rahe, R. H. and Arthur, R. J. (1978). Life changes and illness studies. *Journal of Human Stress*. 4, 3–15.

Redd, W. H. and Andrykowski, M. A. (1982). Behavioural intervention in cancer treatment: Controlling aversive reactions to cancer therapy. *Journal of Consulting and Clinical Psychology*. 43, 595–600.

Reed, G. M., Kemeny, M. E., Taylor, S. E. *et al.* (1994). Realistic acceptance as a predictor of decreased survival time in gay men with AIDS. *Health Psychology*. 13, 299–307.

Reiter, S. and Bendov, D. (1996). The self-concept and quality of life of two groups of learning disabled adults living at home and in groups. *The British Journal of Developmental Disabilities*. 43 (2), 7–135.

Rescorla, R. A. (1967). Pavlovian conditioning and its proper control procedures. *Psychological Review*. 74, 71–80.

Rogers, C. (1951). *Client Centred Therapy*. Boston: Houghton Mifflin.

Rosenhan. D. L. and Seligman, E. P. (1995). *Abnormal Psychology*, 5th Ed. New York: W. H. Norton.

Rosenthal, R. and Jacobson, L. (1968). *Pygmalion in the Classroom: Teacher expectation and pupil's intellectual development*. New York: Holt, Reinhart and Winston.

Ross, L., Amabile, T. M. and Steinmetz, J. L. (1977). Social roles, social control and biases in social perception. *Journal of Personality and Social Psychology*. 35, 485–494.

Rotter, J. B. (1966). Generalised expectancies for the internal versus external control of reinforcement theory. *Psychological Monographs*. 90 (1), 1–28.

Royal College of Physicians and Psychiatrists (1995). *The Psychological Care of Medical Patients: Recognition of need and service provision*. Report by Royal College of Physicians and Psychiatrists, UK.

Ruble, D. N. (1987). The acquisition of self-knowledge: A self-socialisation perspective. In Eisenberg, N. (ed.). *Contemporary Topics in Developmental Psychology*. New York: Wiley-Interscience.

Russell, G. C. (1993). The role of denial in clinical practice. *Journal of Advanced Nursing*, 18, 938–940.

Russell, G. C. (1996). *An Investigation into the Nature of Self-consciousness*. Unpublished master's thesis. University of Plymouth.

Russell, G. C. and Towler, M. (1990). *An Investigation into Factors Causing Delay in Help-seeking with a Community Mental Health Team*. Unpublished research. University of Plymouth.

Salter, M. (1988). *Altered Body Image: The nurse's role*. Chichester: John Wiley.

Sarrafino, E. P. (1994). *Health Psychology: Biopsychosocial interactions*. New York: John Wiley.

Schaefer, C., Coyne, J. C. and Lazarus, R. S. (1981). The health related functions of social support. *Journal of Behavioural Medicine*. 4, 381–486.

Schaie, K. W. (1990). In Birren, J. E. and Schaie, K. W. (Eds). *Handbook of the Psychology of Ageing*. San Diego: Academic Press.

Schalock, R. L., Keith, K. D. and Hoffman, K. (1990). *Quality of Life Standardization Manual*, Hastings, NE: Mid-Nebraska Mental Retardation Services, Inc.

Scheier, M. F. (1976). Self-awareness, self-consciousness and angry aggression. *Journal of Personality*. 44, 627–644.

Scheier, M. F. and Bridges, M. W. (1995). Person variables and health: Personality dispositions and acute psychological states as shared determinants of disease. *Psychosomatic Medicine*. 57, 255–268.

Scheier, M. F. and Carver, C. S. (1985). Optimism, coping and health: Assessment and implications of generalised outcome expectancies. *Health Psychology*. 4, 219–247.

Schlenker, B. R. and Leary, M. R. (1982). Social anxiety and self-presentation: A conceptualisation and model. *Psychological Bulletin*. 92 (3), 641–669.

Schwartz, B. (1984). *Psychology of Learning and Behaviour*. 2nd Ed. New York: Norton.

Scott, L. E. and Glum, G. H. (1984). Coping style and brief treatments for post-surgical pain. *Pain*. 20, 279–291.

Scrambler, G. and Scrambler, A. (1984). The illness iceberg and aspects of consulting behaviour. In Fitzpatrick, R. and Hinton, J. (Eds).*The Experience of Illness*. London: Tavistock.

Seligman, M. E. P. (1971). Phobias and preparedness. *Behaviour Therapy*. 2, 307–320.

Seligman, M. E. P. (1975). *Helplessness: On depression*. San Francisco: Freeman.

Seltzer, A. and Hoffman, B. F. (1980). Drug compliance of the psychiatric patient. *Canadian Family Physician*. 26, 267–280.

Seyle, H. (1979). *The Stress of Life*. (Rev. Ed.). New York: Van Nostrand Reinhold.

Sheldon, W. H. (1954). *Atlas of Man: A guide for somatotyping the adult male of all ages*. New York: Harper and Row.

Shontz, F. G. (1982). Coping with acute health crises. In Millon, T., Green, C. and Meagher, R. (Eds). *Handbook of Clinical Health Psychology*. New York: Plenum.

Shultz, R., Bookwala, J., Knapp, J. *et al.* (1994). Pessimism and mortality in young and old cancer patients. As cited in Scheier, M. F. and Carver, M. W. (1995). Person variables and health. *Psychosomatic Medicine*. 57, 255–268.

Silverman, I. (1964). Self-esteem and differential response to success and failure. *Journal of Abnormal and Social Psychology*. 69, 115–119.

Simmons, M. and Daw, P. (1994). *Stress, Anxiety and Depression: A practical workbook*. Bicester: Winslow Press.

Simmons, R. G., Blyth, D. A. and McKinney, K. L. (1983). The social and psychological effects of puberty on white females. In Brooks-Gunn, J. and Petersen, A. C. (Eds). *Girls and Puberty: Biological and psychosocial perspectives*. New York: Plenum.

Simmons, R. G., Klein, S. D. and Thornton, K. (1973). The family member's decision to be a kidney transplant donor. *Journal of Comparative Family Studies*. 4, 88–115.

Skynner, R. and Cleese, J. (1983). *Families and How to Survive Them*. London: Methuen.

Smith, A. (1995). Measuring quality of life for people with learning disabilities: Is it important, can it be done and who should do it? *Health Psychology Update*. BPS Special Group in Health Psychology. Issue 19, March.

Smith, D. A. (1993). *Stability of Two Quality of Life Measures and Influence of Results in Adults with Learning Disabilities*. Unpublished MSc thesis. University of Leeds.

Smith, T. W. (1992). Hostility and health: Current status of a psychosomatic hypothesis. *Health Psychology*. 11, 139–150.

Snyder, M. (1974). The self-monitoring of expressive behaviour. *Journal of Personality and Social Psychology*. 30, 526–537.

Sroufe, L. A. (1989). Pathways to adaptation and maladaptation: Psychopathology as developmental deviation. In Ciccehti, D. (Ed). *The Emergence of a Discipline. Vol 1*. Hillsdale, NJ: Erlbaum.

Sroufe, L. A. and Fleeson, J. (1986). Attachment and the construction of relationships. In Hartup, W. W. and Rubin, Z. (Eds). *Relationships and Development*. Hillsdale, NJ: Erlbaum.

Staub, E. (1980). *Personality: Basic concepts and current research*. Engelwood Cliffs, NJ: Prentice Hall.

Steptoe, A. and Mathews, A. (1984). *Health Care and Human Behaviour*. London: Academic Press.

Sternberg, R. J. (1985). Beyond IQ: A triarchic theory of human intelligence. *Behavioural and Brain Sciences*. 7, 269–287.

Stockwell, F. (1984). *The Unpopular Patient*. Beckenham: Crook-Helm.

Stone, G. C. (1979). Patient compliance and the role of the expert. *Journal of Social Issues*. 35, 34–59.

Sullivan, H. S. (1953). *The Interpersonal Theory of Psychiatry*. New York: Horton.

Sulls, J. and Mullen, B. (1982). From the cradle to the grave: Comparison and self-evaluation across the lifespan. In Sulls, J. (Ed). *Psychological Perspectives on the Self. Vol. 1*. Hillsdale, NJ: Erlbaum.

Szasz, T. (1975). *The Age of Madness: History of involuntary mental hospitalisation*. London: Routledge and Kegan Paul.

Taylor, S. E. (1983). Adjustment to threatening events: A theory of cognitive adaptation. *American Psychologist*, 38, 1161–1173.

Taylor, S. E. and Brown, J. D. (1988). Illusion and well-being: A social psychological perspective on mental health. *Psychological Bulletin*. 103 (2), 193–210.

Thorndike (1898). Animal intelligence: An experimental study of the associative processes in animals. *Psychological Review* (Monograph supplement). 8 (1) 16.

Trower, P., Gilbert, P. and Sherling, G. (1990). Social anxiety, evolution and self-presentation. In Leitenbreg, H. (Ed). *Handbook of Social and Evaluation Anxiety*. New York: Plenum.

Tuma, A. H. and Maser, J. D. (1985). *Anxiety and Anxiety Disorders*. Hillsdale, NJ: Erlbaum.

Turk, D. C. and Fernandez, E. (1991). Pain: a cognitive-behavioural perspective. In Watson, M. (Ed). *Cancer Patient Care: Psychosocial treatment methods*. Cambridge: BPS Books.

Waterman, A. S. (1995). Identity in the context of adolescent psychology. *New Directions in Child Development*. 30, 5–24,

Watson, D. and Friend, R. (1969). Measurement of social evaluative anxiety. *Journal of Consulting and Clinical Psychology*. 33 (4), 448–457.

Watson, J. B. and Rayner, R. (1928). Conditioned emotional reactions. *Journal of Experimental Psychology*. 3, 1–14.

Watts, F. N. (1979). Behavioural aspects of management of diabetes mellitus. *Behavioural Research and Therapy*. 18, 171–189.

Weiner, B. (1986). *An Attribution Theory of Motivation and Emotion*. New York: Springer Verlag.

Weiss, R. S. (1972). Influence of psychological variables on stress-induced psychology. In Porter, R. and Knight, J. (Eds). *Physiology, Emotion and Psychosomatic Illness*, New York: American Elsevier.

Weiss, R. S. (1993). Loss and recovery. In Stroebe, M. S., Stroebe, W. and Hansson, R. O. (Eds). *A Handbook of Bereavement*. Cambridge: Cambridge University Press.

Whiteman, M. C., Fowkes, R. G. R., Deary, I. J. and Lee, A. J. (1997). Hostility, cigarette smoking and alcohol consumption. *Social Science and Medicine*. 44 (8), 1089–1096.

Wilkinson, S. R. (1988). *The Child's World of Illness: The development of health and illness behaviour*. Cambridge: Cambridge University Press.

Williams, R. B. and Barefoot, J. C. (1988). Coronary prone behaviour. The emerging role of the hostility complex. In Houston, C. K. and Snyder, C. R. (Eds). *Type A Behaviour Pattern, Research, Theory and Intervention.* New York: Wiley.

Wills, T. A. (1982). Downward social comparison: Principles in social psychology. *Psychological Bulletin.* 90, 245–271.

Wolfensberger, W. (1972). *The Principle of Normalisation in Human Services.* Toronto: National Institute of Mental Retardation.

Woods, R. T. and Britton, P. G. (1985). *Clinical Psychology with the Elderly.* Beckenham: Crook-Helm.

Woods, T. (1996). (Ed). *Handbook of Clinical Psychology of Ageing.* Chichester: John Wiley.

Woolf, C. J. (1983). Evidence for a central component of post-injury hypersensitivity. *Nature.* 306, 686–688.

Wortman, C. B. and Silver, R. C. (1989). The myths of coping with loss. *Journal of Consulting and Clinical Psychology.* 57 (3), 349–357.

Wright, B. (1985). Hostility in accident and emergency departments. *Nursing Mirror.* 161 (14), 42–43.

Wright, B. (1986). *Caring in Crisis: A handbook of intervention skills for nurses.* Edinburgh: Churchill Livingstone.

Wright, S. J. (1994). Health-related quality of life: A critical review of the concept and its measurement. In Dauwalder, J. P. (Ed). *Psychology and Promotion of Health.* Seattle: Hogrefe and Huber.

Wykes, T. (1994). *Violence and Health Care Professionals.* London: Chapman Hall.

Yerkes, R. M. and Dodson, J. D. (1908). The relative strength of stimulus to rapidity of habit formation. *Journal of Comparative Neurology and Psychology.* 57 (3), 349–357.

Zaborowski, Z. and Oleszkiewicz, Z. (1988). For a wider study of the context of self-consciousness. *Polish Psychological Bulletin.* 19 (1), 65–75.

Zola, K. I. (1973). Pathways to the doctor – from person to patient. *Social Science and Medicine.* 7, 677–689.

Zola, K. I. (1981). Structural constraints on the doctor–patient relationship. In Eisenberg, L. and Kleinman, M. (Eds). *The Relevance of Social Science for Medicine.* New York: D. Reidel.

Zuckerman, M. (1979). Attribution of success and failure revisited. *Journal of Personality.* 47, 245–283.

Index